WILDERNESS FIRST AID

Steve Donelan

Supporting courses in:

- Basic Wilderness First Aid
- Wilderness First Aid

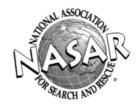

ISBN 978-0-9864440-5-0 (Paperback Edition)

Editing by Steve Donelan and Emily E. James
Cover design and drawings by Evelyn Sinclair, www.gangof1.com
Front cover art adapted from *The Domes of Yosemite* by Albert Bierstadt
Back cover inset photographs by Ben Schifrin, MD, FACEP

Photographs by Ben Schifrin, MD, FACEP; Joanne Clapp Fullager; Ruth McConnell; Mike Cardwell; Oleg Grachev; Linda Garcia; and other sources as credited

Printed and bound in the United States of America
First Printing, 2018

Published by The National Association For Search And Rescue, Inc.
PO Box 232020
Centreville, VA 20120-2020

Visit www.NASAR.org

To my students,
Who are also my teachers

Steve

Contents

Introduction

Wilderness First Aid includes the topics and skills from my *Wilderness Emergency Care* textbook* that are usually taught in wilderness first aid courses. The *WEC* textbook includes many more topics, more thorough explanations, and more advanced skills. But both books are designed to help prepare people for emergencies in wilderness or disaster situations where resources are limited and rapid transport to medical care is not available. They give step-by-step instructions for doing each skill, illustrated with clear drawings or photos.

I hope that you will find this book interesting and enjoyable to read, and that it will help you avoid, prevent and prepare for emergencies by guiding you through mental rehearsals of what can happen and what you can do. As a teacher, I have seen that people learn and remember best if they know the reasons for what they learn. My experience is supported by many studies of skills learning and retention. So I always explain topics, rather than just describe problems and treatments, and I encourage you to make logical and causal connections.

For example, what damage does an injury do, and how does the body react? How does that reaction produce the signs and symptoms that we find when we assess the patient? Similarly, how do the body and brain react to the stress of heat, cold or altitude? Once you've thought through these questions, you should be able to figure out what is going on in an emergency and what to do about it, even if you can't remember exactly what I or another writer recommended.

Medical terms are usually very descriptive and sometimes humorous, but unfortunately they come from Latin or Greek. So I demystify the terms by breaking them down and showing their literal sense (in parentheses and quotes). I put ideas in historical and cultural context because that helps us to understand them. It also reminds us that some ideas may turn out to be wrong, as so many of their predecessors were. So the same process of inquiry and analysis that gives us some confidence in current ideas of wilderness emergency care should prevent us from getting too dogmatic.

In the chapters on injuries, you will find a concise but very thorough guide to bandaging and splinting, including improvised techniques. You will not find many of these in other books. Urban rescuers use standard equipment and their bandages and splints only need to stay on for a short ambulance ride to the hospital. But wilderness rescuers need to be able to improvise with what is available. Their bandages and splints need to stay on while the patient walks, skis, or scrambles out or is evacuated from the backcountry.

Even more important than the physical skills are the mental and social skills of emergency care: Figuring out what the problems are and what is causing them; setting priorities and making a plan; organizing and leading a rescue or working in a team; communicating with the patient and other people on the scene; and coping with the psychological stress of an emergency in yourself and others. You can develop the mental and social skills of emergency care by practicing techniques realistically and doing role-playing scenarios.

However you use this book, I hope it will make your wilderness activities safer and more enjoyable. I also hope that it will prepare you to help yourself and other people in a wilderness emergency or disaster.

Steve Donelan

Wilderness Emergency Care, Third Edition, Revised. National Association for Search and Rescue, 2018.

Chapter 1. Training for Wilderness Emergencies

Urban rescuers face many challenges – technical, physical and psychological. Unless they are involved in a major disaster, however, urban rescuers usually have quick access to medical care, transportation, shelter, supplies and reinforcements. And although they may go into hazardous situations to perform emergency care, these rescuers can usually retreat to safe surroundings.

In the wilderness or a disaster situation, you can count on none of these advantages. You may have to care for patients for many hours during bivouacs or strenuous evacuations. Your shelter and supplies will be what you have with you or can improvise, and reinforcements may be long in coming. With limited resources, you must protect your patients and yourself against weather and other environmental hazards. What kind of training prepares you for wilderness emergencies or major disasters?

Before you can take care of others, you must first learn the survival skills needed to take care of yourself in the wilderness. These skills include knowing what to carry and to wear to survive the worst possible conditions. You should learn how the body interacts with environmental stresses such as heat, cold and altitude; and how clothing and shelter can control this interaction. You should also practice first aid skills, such as bandaging and splinting, on yourself as well as on others because you may have to treat your own injuries.

Psychological aspects of first aid

Any serious emergency can make first aiders as well as victims feel that they are losing control of events. In the wilderness, the strange surroundings, exposure, and insidious effects of environmental stress on the brain all can combine to induce fear, despair or apathy. You can begin training yourself to cope with these stresses by understanding them.

Everyone is susceptible to stress. Behavior that denies or evades the reality of an unpleasant situation is common. This behavior may range from unrealistic assessments or plans to apathy or withdrawal. Some may react by blaming themselves or others in the group. Others may have sensory disturbances like tunnel vision or muffled hearing.

By recognizing these behavioral problems as signs of emergency stress, you can avoid being pulled into unproductive emotional responses. When causes of the stress are physical, simple physical measures, such as rehydration, energy food, and protection from the elements, can have major psychological benefits. Productive action also gives people a sense of regaining control. Reasoning with the unrealistic and reassuring the fearful may help, but tactful redirection to useful tasks is often more effective therapy.

Every serious injury or illness has psychological effects. Patients may be locked into an internal conversation about pain or fear. As a first aider, you need to join in this conversation and redirect it to what you and the patient can do, together, to help. Those who are seriously ill or injured are often in a highly suggestible state, so what you say and how you say it can influence autonomic nervous system functions, positively or negatively. These functions include pulse, blood pressure, respiration, and the inflammatory response to an injury. Even in a positive context, scare words like "die" or "bleeding" can have a negative effect. Instead, use only positive or neutral words (and never describe the injuries) when a patient can hear; but always tell the truth.

If a patient asks about his or her injuries, acknowledge the problem in neutral terms, then redirect the conversation to what you can do to help. For example, if a patient asks "Is my leg broken?' you can say "There is an injury, but let's put a splint on it, and tell me if that makes it more comfortable."

Injury or illness can suppress or alter body language and facial expression as well as speech. While rescuers usually understand this in theory, the absent or altered signals can still make it hard for them to communicate with patients. Practicing a splint on a partner who is joking and moving the supposedly injured limb about freely does not prepare you to treat someone with a real fracture. So you should always get into the role of first aider or patient when practicing skills and behave realistically.

Communication and teamwork

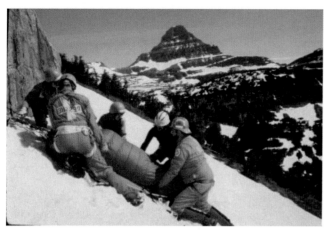

Photo courtesy of Ben Schifrin, MD

One of the hardest lessons to learn in emergency care is that democracy does not work at an accident scene. When acting as leader, you learn to plan ahead and give unambiguous directions. As a member of the team, you learn to listen to the leader, talk as little as possible, and address questions or suggestions to the leader. Cross discussions cut the lines of leadership. It is also important that only one rescuer talk to each patient. When you play the role of patient in class, you learn how disorienting it is to have several voices competing for your already distracted attention.

Legal and ethical aspects

Before providing emergency care, you need the **consent** of the patient. You should also explain what you want to do so that the patient understands the **risks** (if any) – that makes it **informed consent**. If the patient is (or becomes) unresponsive, that is **implied consent**. The law presumes that anyone who cannot respond needs help. When treating a **minor**, you should get permission from any parent or legal guardian present, but you should also persuade the child to let you help.

When you provide emergency care, your legal status depends on whether you have a **duty to act**. Medical professionals who are on the job or at their place of employment where emergency care is normally provided always have a duty to act in an emergency, even if they are not on shift. In some countries, any bystander has a legal duty to provide assistance in an emergency (provided that it is safe to do so) but not in the United States. Even in the United

States, however, the law recognizes a duty to aid and protect anyone in a relationship of **dependence**, which would include participants of an organized wilderness trip, and imply that the leader has a duty to act.

Anyone with a duty to act is held to a **standard of care** depending on level of training and **scope of practice**; and failure to meet that standard on duty is **negligence**. To prove negligence, an attorney has to prove all four elements:

- The care provider had a **duty to act**.
- There was a **breach** of duty, meaning that the provider failed to do something he or she should have done or did something NOT in the provider's scope of practice.
- That act or omission was the **cause**
- of **harm** to the patient.

Every state in the United States has a **Good Samaritan Law** to encourage people who do not have a duty to act to help in an emergency. For example, the California law says: "No person who in good faith, and not for compensation, renders emergency medical or nonmedical care at the scene of an emergency shall be liable for any civil damages resulting from any act or omission." *California Health and Safety Code 1799.102(a)*.

The story of the Good Samaritan is told in Luke 10:30-37. A Jewish traveler was wounded by thieves, who stripped him and left him lying on the road, half dead. Two other Jewish travelers saw him, but "passed by on the other side." Then a Samaritan (a sect very hostile to the Jews in Biblical times) "had compassion on him, and bound up his wounds, pouring in oil and wine, and set him on his own beast, and brought him to an inn, and took care of him." *King James Version*

If you choose to act as a Good Samaritan, remember that the law has four elements, and that all four must be observed for the law to apply:

- You do NOT have a duty to act.
- You do emergency care.
- It is at the emergency scene.
- You do NOT expect or accept any compensation.

Once you choose to begin care as a Good Samaritan, you have a legal as well as moral obligation to continue care until relieved by someone of equal or greater training. Otherwise, you could be accused of **abandonment**. Moreover, in a serious wilderness accident, your situation could still be an emergency scene until the patient was evacuated to safety, though going out for help (if there is no other option) would be a necessary part of wilderness emergency care, and not abandonment.

In describing the standard of care expected from a Good Samaritan, the phrase "what any reasonable and prudent adult would do" is common. For wilderness emergencies, this translates into doing what you have been trained to do competently.

Volunteer outings leaders for organizations like the Sierra Club and Scouts do have a duty to act if someone in their group needs help. So they are not covered by a Good Samaritan Act. But a federal law, the **Volunteer Protection Act of 1997** (Public Law 105-19) is meant to protect volunteers for non-profit organizations against frivolous lawsuits, which were discouraging people from volunteering. However, it applies only to volunteers who were acting "within the scope of the volunteer's responsibilities" which would be defined by the organization for which they volunteer. Volunteers must also be "properly licensed, certified, or authorized by the appropriate authorities for the activities or practice in the state for which the harm occurred". Again, the volunteers' organization should determine what certifications or licenses are needed for the activity that the volunteers lead. The act does not apply to volunteers operating a vehicle, however, or to someone guilty of gross negligence.

Injuries

Slides can be invaluable, especially if they show the accident scene (mechanism of injury) and close-ups of injuries (damage done). But the effect of gruesome injuries can be amplified if you are locked into a spectator role, which leaves you with nothing to do but react to the scene emotionally or try to escape. Avoid this problem by asking yourself and visualizing how to treat each injury.

In a real accident, taking positive action to help the victims redirects the mind, at least during the scene. That is why you must practice until basic skills become reflexive. These reflexes can carry you through the first emotional impact of the scene. Also, learning how injuries damage the body and affect the vital systems trains you in whole-accident response, rather than single-skill tunnel vision. You learn to treat the patient first and the injury second.

Sudden illness, trauma, and shock

Illness kills in two ways: by disrupting vital systems and by diminishing the victim's ability to avoid accidents. In working through accident scenarios, you should check for medical causes, especially if the accident does not otherwise make sense. By including false leads among the causes, instructors train students to consider all the evidence. For example, diabetes can mimic the effects of alcohol abuse.

Getting the history of the present illness is akin to reconstructing the mechanism of an injury. In both cases, you are finding causal connections that converge to a damaging event. Both lines of inquiry can uncover problems that you would otherwise have missed. Any problem that interferes with the delivery of oxygen to the vital organs usually has first priority, and anticipating problems may give you the margin needed to save lives.

Begin by looking at the systems that deliver oxygen to the tissues: airways, lungs, pump, pipes, fluid, and signals that control them. Then you can work out what happens when different parts of the system are damaged or disrupted. For example, what effects can chest injuries have on breathing? How can the circulatory system compensate for loss of blood? What injuries can interrupt signals from the brain to the respiratory or circulatory system? A similar approach can be used to learn about sudden illness. Once you understand how an injury or illness affects different parts of the body, or disrupts vital systems, you can work out what signs and symptoms will be produced.

Environmental stress

When the body's internal environment is pushed to extremes, we need to re-examine our understanding of vital processes and emergency procedures. Until the 1960s, for instance, High Altitude Pulmonary Edema (HAPE) was routinely diagnosed as pneumonia and treated with antibiotics. Victims who were not promptly brought down to lower elevations often died. People have also died of undiagnosed heat stroke because, contrary to what the textbooks said, their skins were still pale and sweaty. We learn to begin CPR if we find no pulse, but what about a victim in deep hypothermia, who may have an impalpable pulse?

These examples teach us to focus on what is happening to the vital systems, just as with sudden illness. Shortage of oxygen during an ascent can have many unpleasant effects, including headache and nausea. However, if the respiratory or central nervous system is disrupted, then the victim needs to relieve the stress on the system by descending.

For instance, if one climber always remains fatigued and short of breath after resting, when others are ready to go on, then we should suspect HAPE. We needn't wait until we hear fluid gurgling in the lungs or the victim starts coughing up pink sputum. Similarly, if someone's mental functions and balance are seriously impaired after exposure to altitude, we should suspect High Altitude Cerebral Edema.

Heat exhaustion often looks like compensated, hypovolemic shock. In both conditions, blood volume is down because of fluid loss, and circulation is withdrawn from the skin and skeletal muscles. Hence the pulse (especially in the wrist) is usually weak, and the heart compensates for low stroke volume by speeding up. Skin is pale, cool and clammy.

The victim usually feels nauseated as well as weak, because circulation to the digestive system is a low priority for the body. Comparing heat exhaustion with shock, and working out the differences of mechanism and treatment, illuminate the circulatory system's two main functions – delivery, especially of oxygen, and heat transfer.

In heat stroke, there is a conflict between these functions since carrying excess heat to the skin takes circulation away from vital organs. If heat accumulates in the body, the temperature in the vital organs can get dangerously high even if the victim is still pale and sweating. In a conscious victim, irrational behavior is a more reliable danger signal than skin appearance, because the brain is very sensitive to temperature.

Behavioral changes may also be the first warning of hypothermia. Listing brain functions that become impaired as body temperature goes down (from reasoning to coordination to balance) yields a level of responsiveness table familiar from other contexts. Thinking about how to rewarm a hypothermia victim reminds us of how the body produces heat and controls temperature.

The controversy about doing CPR on a hypothermic victim with no perceptible vital signs illustrates an important principle of first aid instruction. Even established procedures like CPR, which instructors drill into students, are based on assumptions about the situation. When variables are introduced, as often happens in the wilderness, we may need to make judgments about procedures that we would do automatically elsewhere. If you start CPR, will it be physically possible to continue CPR during evacuation? Can you even maintain the victim's temperature while doing CPR, much less rewarm? How close are you to your own margin of survival? Working through hypothetical situations trains you to take nothing for granted in a wilderness emergency.

Biological hazards

Although snakes and bears are more dramatic classroom topics, arthropods and microorganisms cause far more problems. All wild water may be contaminated, and there is no perfect way to disinfect it. Boiling water requires fuel and time. Ceramic filters can crack if dropped or allowed to freeze when wet. Paper filters must be replaced when they clog up. Neither filter is certain to take out viruses. No chemical is completely reliable, and chemical disinfection is hindered by sediment or cold water.

There is much folklore and misinformation about bugs and snakes. Slash and suck snakebite kits, for instance, were sold for many years, and an article in 1991 advised shocking victims with DC current to "devitalize" snake venom. Also there is much folklore about insect repellents. Outdoor magazines have advertised everything from vitamin B pills to ultrasound generators. Yet the only repellents that have any effect in laboratory tests are chemicals like DEET, which appear to jam sense receptors of some insects.

Most wild animals, from wasps to bears, will not attack if we avoid provoking them. Staying out of their way requires that we understand something about their behavior and habitats. Blood-feeding arthropods like ticks and mosquitoes may seek us out, but humans are aberrant hosts for most of them. Abnormal behavior in wild mammals (e.g., friendliness) may be a sign of rabies. You need to educate yourself about the actual biological hazards where you will be going, and get up-to-date information on coping with possible damage.

Navigating the body

In order to discuss and document injuries and medical problems, we need terms for directions on the human body and movements. Directional terms come in pairs. **Superior** means toward the head; **inferior** toward the feet. **Anterior** means toward the front of the body; **posterior** means toward the rear. **Medial** means toward the midline of the body; **lateral** away from the midline. So, for example, the nose is superior to the mouth, medial to the eyes, and anterior to the ears. For navigating the arms and legs, we need two more terms: proximal and distal. **Proximal** means closer to the heart; **distal** means further away from the heart. For example, the elbow is distal to the shoulder, but proximal to the wrist. When we check distal nerve functions and signs of circulation, we mean distal to an injury, because we want to know if the injury is affecting circulation or nerve functions. For purposes of anatomical description, we assume that the body is in the anatomical position: standing with arms at the sides, palms forward.

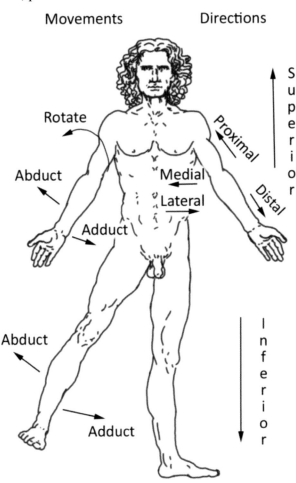

From that position, the arms and legs can **abduct** (move away from the midline of the body) or **adduct** (move toward the midline of the body). They can also **rotate**. Joints in the body and limbs also enable us to **flex** and **extend**, as the side view shows. Solid arrows point in the direction a part of a limb or the body moves when it flexes. Hollow arrows point in the direction a part of a limb or the body moves when it extends. Like abduct and adduct, flex and extend refer to opposite movements. Another way to think of it is that when we flex every part of the body, we are moving into the fetal position. When we extend every part of the body, we are moving away from the fetal position. The corresponding movements of the foot, however, are called dorsiflex and plantarflex, from the Latin *planta* "sole of the foot" and *dorsum* "back of the foot".

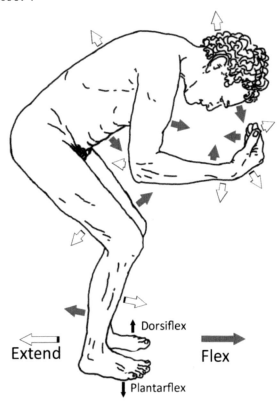

Using these terms for body directions and movements, we can describe the location of an injury or sign (such as swelling or deformity), a patient's position (e.g. arms flexed), and what an injured patient can and cannot do, e.g. can flex an injured forearm but not rotate it. These terms are also part of the vocabulary we need in order to learn about human anatomy.

Chapter 2. Patient Assessment

To treat a patient effectively, you first need to find the problems and set priorities. This process of assessment begins as you approach the scene. In what position is the patient? How does he or she appear? Are there clues on the scene to the mechanism of injury? Are there hazards that would make it dangerous to approach? Urgent problems (such as severe bleeding) that you need to deal with immediately? Is the patient responding? Does the patient look at you spontaneously or only when you give a voice or touch stimulus? Is the patient oriented to identity, place, and time, and event (able to describe what happened?)

If the patient accepts your offer to help, you have two ways of finding the problems: physical examination and asking questions. With a responsive patient, however, both ways are forms of communication. You may see an open wound or deformed limb immediately, but the patient's response to your physical exam can alert you to other, less obvious injuries. A patient may be expressing pain or discomfort with body language. For example, someone having a heart attack may be clutching his or her chest and wincing; and someone with an injury may be guarding and protecting it.

Patients who are not responding vocally may still respond by flinching, grimacing, guarding or withdrawing from your touch. In a responsive patient, even the pulse may change depending on whether you reassure or cause anxiety. Breathing may change if the patient becomes aware that you are observing it. Communication skills in assessment, therefore, include more than getting and giving information vocally. You also need to understand responses with the eyes or body, and the effects that your own words, body language, and manner may have on the patient.

Observation, especially visual, includes interpretation. We tend to see what we expect to see and often overlook what we do not expect. Practicing patient assessment in a standard way should link problem-finding techniques with understanding of the problems, so that you observe intelligently.

If the **mechanism of injury** (MOI) or **nature of illness** (NOI) is minor, with no sign of more serious problems, you will usually need to do only a focused assessment. For example, if someone twists an ankle, is the swelling interfering with circulation and nerve function in the foot? And in a wilderness situation, can the patient still walk? But if the mechanism of injury was a hard impact from a fall or collision, you should do a complete assessment, especially if the accident may have been caused by a medical problem. Similarly, any medical condition that is affecting vital signs can develop into an emergency, or cause an accident by reducing mental and physical efficiency.

Patient assessment includes vital signs, medical history, and head to toe exam. **Vital signs** are observable measures of vital functions. For example, rate, depth, and apparent effort of breathing are measures of how well the respiratory system is working. Rate and strength of pulses in arteries that we can feel just under the skin are measures of how well the circulatory system is working. Skin color and temperature help you evaluate both respiratory and circulatory system function. How the patient responds to questions helps you evaluate brain function. **Medical history** should include any medical problems, previous injuries, or medications that could affect the patient's condition or your treatment. **Head to toe exam** should be thorough and systematic.

Checking breathing and pulse

For an unresponsive patient with no signs of breathing, the mnemonic (from the 2015 Guidelines published by the American Heart Association) is **CAB** (**Circulation, Airway, Breathing**), which means to start chest compressions if an unresponsive patient has no pulse, then open the airway and ventilate. But for patients who are breathing, especially those with injuries, we still use the old mnemonic: ABCs for **Airway, Breathing**, and **Circulation** (including **severe** bleeding). Even a patient who is breathing may not be breathing adequately, and that is still a priority.

If the patient is breathing, you need to learn more about it and other vital signs. Skin signs (color, temperature, turgor or skin tension, moist or dry) can be checked as part of the head-to-toe along with the appearance of the eyes.

When you push gently on an artery with your fingertips, you can feel and time the surges of blood pushed out by contractions of the left ventricle of the heart. For an **unresponsive** adult or child, the carotid pulse is the easiest to find because the artery is big and close to the heart. Slide two or three fingertips between the trachea (Greek *traxus* "rough" because of its corrugated structure) and the slanting strap muscle of the neck just below the jaw. Always take the pulse on your side of the patient's neck. If you reach across the trachea (the mugger's grip) your action may be misunderstood, and you may squeeze the trachea. On an **infant**, whose neck is short and small, find the pulse on the **brachial artery** where it passes over the bone on the inside of the upper arm.

With a **responsive** adult or child, check the radial pulse at the wrist, because poking fingers into the neck would be uncomfortable for the patient. The radial artery can be felt at the base of the thumb, in the groove between the bony edge of the wrist and the tendon that enables you to flex your index finger. If you cannot feel the pulse, press a bit harder with the downstream finger (closest to the thumb) to dam up the blood under the upstream fingers and create a stronger pulse. Count for 30 seconds and multiply by two to get the rate per minute.

What is a normal pulse? That depends on many factors including age. An infant's pulse may be as high as 160 per minute, twice as fast as an adult's. Pregnant women at term may have a resting pulse of up to 100. An adult marathon runner may have a resting pulse of 50. Even if you're not sure what is normal for a patient, an increase in resting pulse or increase in pulse when the patient sits or stands is usually a sign of trouble.

In a responsive patient, take the radial pulse for 30 seconds; then watch and feel chest movement for 30 seconds. Pulse can be described in terms of its rate, strength, and rhythm. Breathing can be described in terms of its rate, depth, and rhythm. For an adult at rest, a breathing rate of 12 to 20 per minute is considered normal. Breathing may also be easy or labored, quiet or noisy. It may hurt to breathe deeply. Breathing may be unequal in the two sides of the chest, because of chest injury or problems with one lung. In an adult, breathing from the diaphragm alone, with no chest motion, may be a sign of cervical spine injury. In infants and toddlers, however, belly breathing (from the diaphragm alone) is normal because the intercostal muscles of the rib cage are undeveloped.

Capillary refill is a quick test of local circulation. Press on a nail bed (or skin if the patient is wearing nail polish) and see how long it takes for the capillaries to pink it out with blood again. Two seconds is about normal. In cold weather, however, circulation to the extremities is usually reduced. Compensation for hypovolemic shock also includes withdrawing blood from the extremities, so you should do the capillary refill test on the forehead as well as the nail beds, and compare the results. With very dark-skinned people, you will not be able to blanch the forehead, but gums and conjunctiva (inside the eyelids) on an unresponsive patient may be visibly pale and bloodless.

Pulse games

Practice counting the pulse in groups of three, with two people each taking one wrist of the third. After counting silently for 30 seconds, the two pulse-takers compare results. Another exercise is to stand behind your partner and find the radial pulse in the raised left arm with your left hand; then grip the upper arm from below in about the middle, with your right hand, pressing on the brachial artery with the flats of your fingers. You will feel the radial pulse disappear.

Level Of Responsiveness

Level of responsiveness (LOR) includes vocal, eye, and motor response. A simple mnemonic for LOR is **AVPU**: **Alert**; responds to **Vocal** stimuli; responds to **Pain** stimuli (e.g., a pinch); and **Unresponsive**.

Getting the medical history

The SAMPLE mnemonic will guide you through the questions you should ask to get the patient's history.

• S stands for Signs and **Symptoms**. What signs of injury or medical problems do you observe (i.e., see, feel, hear, smell)? What symptoms does the patient describe (e.g., pain, discomfort, tingling, numbness)?

• A stands for **Allergies**. Ask whether the patient is allergic to anything, including medications, latex, foods, beestings, pollen, etc.

• M stands for **Medications**. Is the patient taking any? For what? When? Does he or she need to take a medication? Can you assist?

- P stands for **Pertinent** medical history, including Pregnancy. Give examples of medical problems to make sure that the patient understands the question.
- L stands for **Last** oral intake (food, water) and output (urination). When?
- E stands for **Events** leading up to the emergency. If it was a medical problem, what brought it on? If it was an accident, reconstruct the mechanism from clues at the scene and testimony from the patient and bystanders. Find out if a medical or environmental problem helped cause the accident, e.g. hypoglycemia, heat, cold, altitude, seizure, etc.

Is a known disease causing the present problem? If so, what led up to it? Are you finding any signs and symptoms that suggest a medical problem?

Patients' reaction to pain depends on their temperament, and may be affected by the impression you make. **Pain** can be described in terms of its quality, quantity, location, timing, setting and whether anything changes it. For example, a crushing pain in the chest is typical of a heart attack, whereas a sharp pain in the chest may be a blood clot in the lungs (pulmonary embolism).

Throbbing describes pain intensified by the pulse. The surge of blood through the arteries that increases blood pressure makes it worse. A pain may be localized or a diffuse ache. It may radiate (as pain from a heart attack often does) or even be referred (felt in another location). Ask when the pain began, in what circumstances, whether it is constant or intermittent, whether anything makes it better or worse, and whether the patient has done anything to relieve the pain.

Checklist: Vital signs and history

HI
Hazards? Victims? Mechanism of injury/illness? Assess the scene and patient's appearance as you approach.
Introduce yourself and offer to help.

ABCs in the wilderness (EMS *NOT* available)
If the patient (with injuries) does not respond, check:
- **Airway**: No sign of breathing? Open the airway.
- **Breathing**? If not, start rescue breathing.
- **Circulation**: If no pulse, start CPR.
- **Serious** bleeding? Stop the leak.

Spinal/head injury possible? Ask:
- Did you hit your head?
- Did you lose consciousness?
- Any pain or discomfort in your head, neck or back?

SAMPLE history
Ask about:
- **Symptoms** (Pain? Discomfort? Nausea?).
- **Allergies**: To what? Medications? Latex? Bee stings? Foods?
- **Medications**: Taking any? For what? Need to take? Indications of substance abuse?
- **Pertinent** medical history, including pregnancy. Give examples of possible medical problems.
- **Last** oral intake (When? What?) and output.
- **Events** leading up to the accident: Mechanism of injury? Medical/environmental factors?

PAIN
Where? Since when? Quality (sharp? dull?) How much (scale of 1 to 10)? What makes it better or worse?

LOR (Level Of Responsiveness)
Check the patient's level of responsiveness: The patient may respond with the eyes, speech, or body movement (Glasgow Coma Scale). **Oriented** to identity, place, time, event? Is the LOR changing?

PULSE and BREATHING
Check the **radial pulse** 30 seconds in a responsive patient and multiply by 2 to get the rate per minute. Then while pretending you are still checking the pulse, check **breathing** for 30 seconds: rate, depth, rhythm, easy/labored, noise, etc. Check blood pressure and breath sounds if you have the equipment.

SKIN SIGNS
Check the skin on the forehead with the back of your hand: hot or cool, sweaty or dry, elastic or loose when pinched? In a dark-skinned patient, check color in gums. If the patient is unresponsive, check inside the peeled-back eyelid.

Head-to-toe exam

Photos courtesy of Ruth McConnell

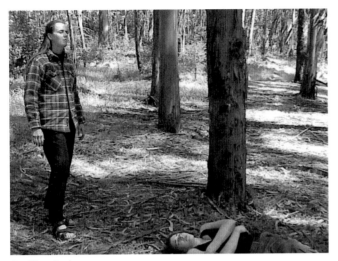

1. Check the scene.

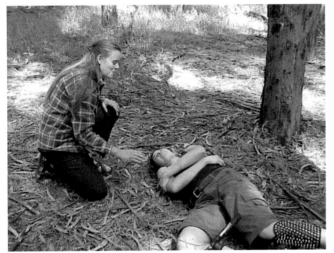

2. Check responsiveness. Ask what happened, introduce yourself and offer to help.

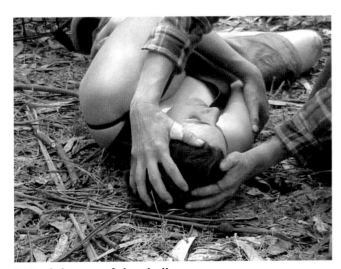

3. Feel the top of the skull.

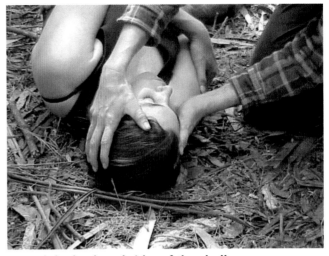

4. Feel the back and sides of the skull

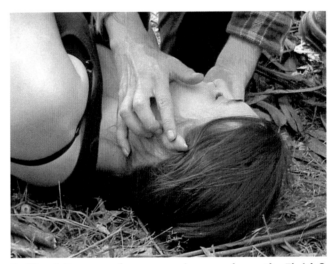

5. Check the ears, face, nose, jaw, and mouth: Fluids? Bruising?

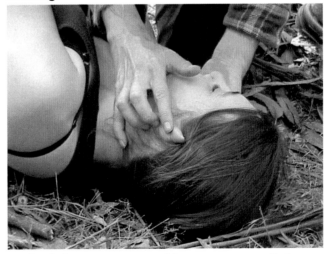

6. Check for raccoon eyes. Also compare pupil size and shape, check light response and eye movement.

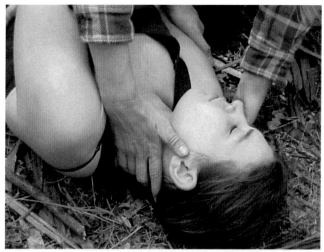

7. Check the facial bones, jaw, and neck. Feel the cervical vertebrae for deformity and "ouches."

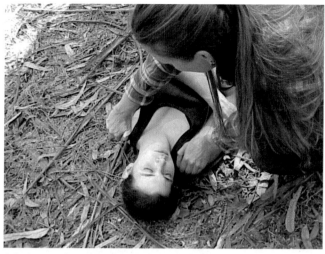

10. Press the shoulders downward.

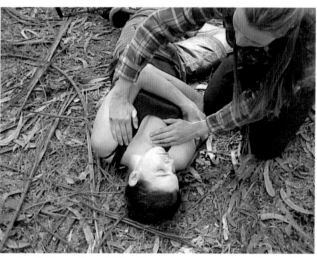

8. Feel each clavicle from one end to the other.

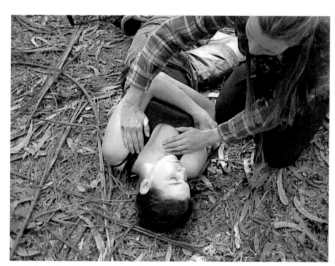

11. Feel the sternum (breast bone) inch by inch. Watch for signs of pain.

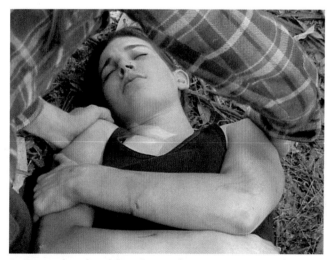

9. Press the shoulders inward.

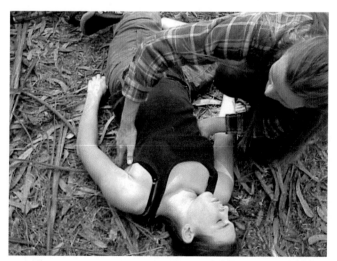

12. Press in on the rib cage. Ask the patient to take a deep breath and point to where it hurts.

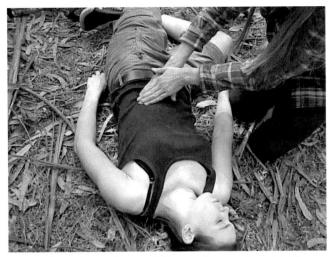

13. Feel each quadrant of the abdomen for rigidity, distension or signs of tenderness.

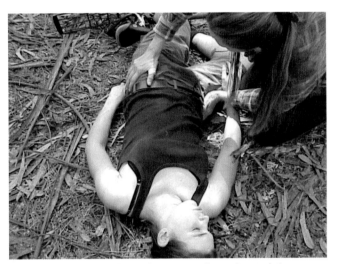

14. Press inward, then downward on the pelvis.

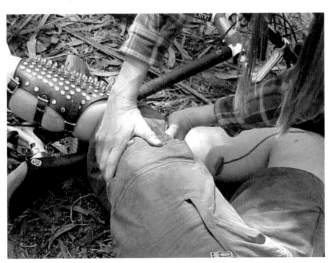

15. Check each leg for deformity and tenderness, working around where the patient says it hurts.

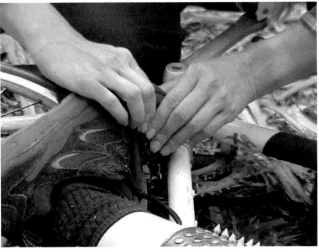

16. Ask, "which toe am I pressing?" "Can you wiggle your toes?"

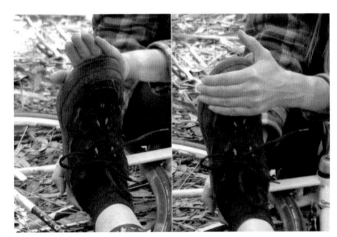

17. Ask the patient to press down and up on your hand with her foot.

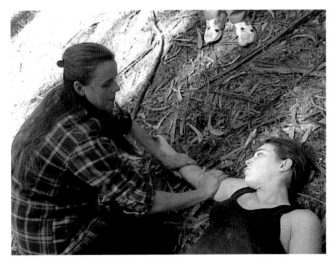

18. Feel each arm for deformities and "ouches."

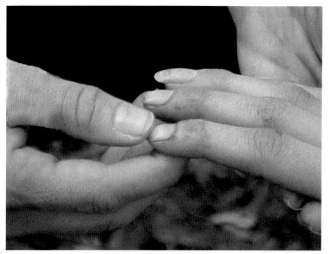

19. Check capillary refill and other signs of circulation (skin color, temperature) in the fingers.

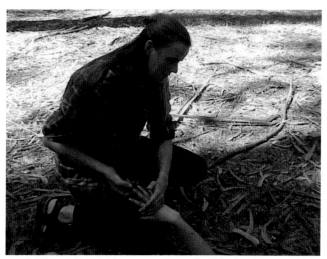

20. Ask "Which finger am I touching? Wiggle your fingers?"

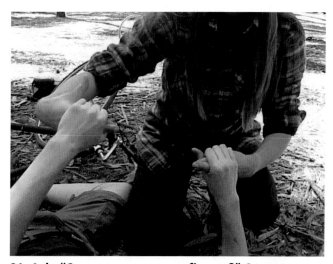

21. Ask, "Can you squeeze my fingers?" Compare strength in the patient's two hands.

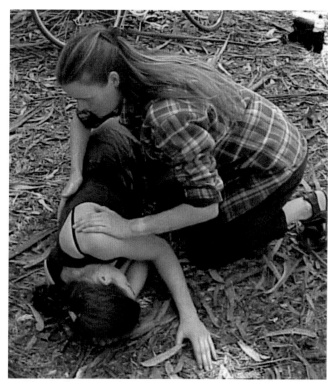

22. If the patient shows no sign of spinal injury, roll her towards you and check the back for injuries.

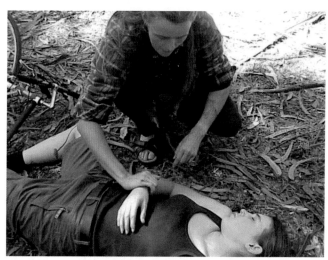

23. Check the radial pulse for 30 seconds. Then (without telling the patient), count breaths for 30 seconds. Multiply by 4 to get the rate per minute. Check blood pressure and breath sounds if you have the equipment.

Checklist: Head-to-toe exam

Always go to skin if necessary to find out what the injury is. If clothing cannot be unbuttoned or unzipped, use a seam ripper or shears.

HEAD

Scalp: Look for bleeding or open wounds.
Skull: If no obvious wound, feel for depressions.
Forehead: Hot? Cold? Moist? Feel with backs of fingers. Turgor? Pinch the skin.
Pupils: Dilated? Constricted? Unequal? Glazed? Light response? Contact lenses?
Eyes: Hold the head: "How many fingers? Follow the fingers." Raccoon eyes?
Nose: Broken? Clear or blood-tinged fluid draining?
Facial bones: Deformity? Bruising? Point tenderness?
Ears: Bruises behind (Battle's sign)? Clear or blood-tinged fluid draining? Capture patch of bloody fluid on white cloth (halo or ring test).
Jaw: "Can you open it? Wiggle it from side to side?"
Tongue: "Can you stick it out?" Straight or twisted?
Mouth Bleeding? Foreign objects? Check alignment of teeth. Missing or false teeth?
Breath: Odor?

NECK

Trachea Deviated? Check for chest/lung injury.
Muscles: Tensed? Check for other signs of respiratory distress/disease.
Veins: Distended? Suspect right heart failure.
Stoma? Look for small hole or tube near base of neck.
Cervical spine: Feel for point tenderness & deformity.
Medic alert tag: On chain around neck?

CHEST & SHOULDERS

Clavicles: Feel for point tenderness & deformity.
Shoulders: Press in, then back. Any pain?
Sternum: Feel for point tenderness & deformity.
Rib cage: Gently press in with both hands as victim takes a deep breath. Pain? Where?
Motion of chest: Asymmetrical? Paradoxical? Guarding? Diaphragm or chest movement only?

ABDOMEN

Look: Bleeding? Wounds? Bruising? Guarding? Distended?
Feel (one prod per quad): Rigidity? Distension? Pain?

SPINE

Feel as much as you can without moving the patient. Deformity?
Watch the patient's face and **listen** for an "Ouch!"- point tenderness?

PELVIS

Look and **smell** for incontinence (loss of bowel &/or bladder control).
Pelvic bones: Press in, then down. Any pain?

LEGS

Look: Bleeding? Bruising? Angulation? Deformity?
Feel down each leg with both hands, firmly. Pain? Point tenderness?

FEET

Look & feel. Signs of injuries in legs or feet? Check
Circulation: Check color, warmth, capillary refill (press nail beds).
Pulse: Posterior tibial (behind inside ankle knob) & dorsalis pedis (top of foot). Equal in both feet?
Sensation: "Which toe am I touching?" Make sure patient can't see it.
Movement: "Can you wiggle your toes?"
Strength: "Can you press up, down against my hand?"

ARMS

Look: Bleeding? Swelling? Deformity? Medic alert bracelet?
Feel down each arm with both hands, firmly. Pain? Point tenderness?
Pulse : Radial (wrist, near base of thumb). Equal in both wrists?

HANDS

Signs of injury in legs or feet? If so, check
Functions: Sensation, finger movement, strength.
Circulation: Check color, warmth, capillary refill.

BACK

Look: Bleeding? Bruising? Deformity?
Feel: Deformity? Point tenderness in spine?

Format for an accident report

Name, Age and Sex of the patient
Chief Complaint: What bothers the patient most?
Vital Signs should include LOR, pulse, breathing, and skin signs Record the results and times, and note any changes.
SAMPLE history
- **Symptoms**: Pain? Discomfort? Vertigo?
- **Allergies**: To medications, latex, foods, beestings, pollen, etc.?
- **Medications**: Prescribed? For what? Over the counter? Herbal/alternative? Last taken?
- **Pertinent** medical history: Medical problems? Past injuries? Pregnant?
- **Last** oral intake: Food or drink, including alcohol.
- **Events** leading up to the emergency: Medical? Environmental? Physical (e.g., fall, collision)? Reconstruct **mechanism of injury** (MOI).

Physical Exam
- General Appearance, body position, apparent level of distress.
- Head-To-Toe Exam: What observable signs of injuries or medical problems did you find? What pain or discomfort did the patient express with body language?

Treatment: Briefly report what you did.

Oral report

When you turn over care of the patient, tell the new care giver what he or she needs to know immediately about the patient. Organize what you observed and were told into categories: patient's name, age, and general appearance; chief complaint; SAMPLE history; vital signs; injuries; treatment. It should take you no more than one minute to present the facts, with no narrative or unnecessary words.

Example: "This is John Doe. He's 28 years old. John was found sitting at the base of a boulder and complained of pain in his right ankle. He is alert and oriented times 4, pulse 70, and respirations 12.He reports no other symptoms besides pain, denies any allergies; carries an inhaler for asthma, but denies any other medical problems; had an energy bar for lunch; fell when he was bouldering and injured his ankle. We splinted it and carried him out."

Patients with disabilities

Many people with sensory, physical, or developmental disabilities engage in outdoor activities. On the ski slopes, you may see blind skiers with guides ahead of them calling the turns, one-legged skiers on monoskis, and paraplegics in ski sleds. People with physical disabilities also do other outdoor activities, such as hiking and mountain climbing.

Over six million people in the United States have visual disabilities, even with glasses; and over one million are **legally blind**, with vision of 20/200 or worse. About one million people in the United States are functionally **deaf**, and nearly ten million are hard of hearing. **American Sign Language** (ASL) is the third most used native language in the United States, after English and Spanish.

Developmental disabilities can affect mental, sensory or motor functions. Traumatic brain injury can cause similar loss of function.

Patients with impaired motor functions may be using canes or walkers, or be in wheelchairs. They may have impaired speech, but that does not necessarily mean their intelligence is affected. Moreover, most people with disabilities value their independence, and must be treated with respect. So it is important to communicate clearly and make sure you have their permission.

Assessing the deaf and blind

Very few deaf people can read lips, especially the lips of strangers. So unless you know their language (ASL), you need to communicate with them in writing, and keep it simple. Those who were born deaf, or went deaf at an early age, tend to have a low reading level because it is hard to learn how to read without phonetics. You also need to be careful to stay within deaf patients' sight, so that they know what you are doing. Two web sites can help you learn ASL signs for communicating with the deaf: www.signingsavvy.com and www.lifeprint.com. Both web sites have video dictionaries of ASL.

If you need to help a blind person walk to safety, offer your arm or shoulder and let the patient hold it. Describe the terrain ahead. When assessing blind patients, tell them exactly what you are going to do before you touch them, and what you are doing as you proceed. Although blind people often learn to compensate with their other senses, any serious injury or medical problem disrupts the feeling of control over one's own life. Good communication, and giving the patient choices whenever it is possible, can help restore that feeling of control.

Recovery position

A patient who is unresponsive but breathing, and has no indications of spinal injury, should usually be left in the recovery (left lateral) position. A supine patient who feels nauseated should also be rolled into this position to protect the airway. Since the stomach is on the left side of the body, the recovery position keeps stomach contents below the esophagus; and vomit is less likely to be aspirated into the lungs.

Moving a patient into recovery position

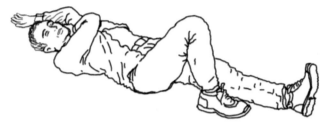

Raise the right knee, lay the left arm alongside the head, and place the right hand on the left shoulder.

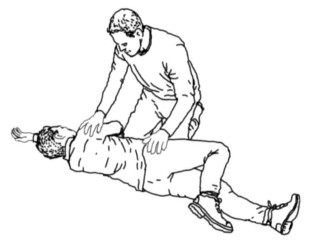

Grip shoulder and hip, and roll the patient towards you onto his side.

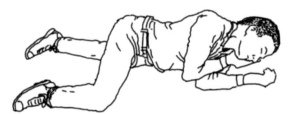

The patient's right knee and right elbow keep him in a stable position that helps to protect the airway.

Chapter 3. Environmental hazards
Effects of heat, cold, altitude, sunlight, and lightning strike

Heat

Our cells process glucose for energy, but 75% of that energy is heat. If we do not get rid of excess heat fast enough, it cooks the brain and other vital organs. How does the body dump excess heat? First, the blood must carry heat from the vital organs and muscles to the skin. Fluid flowing from a heat source to cooler surroundings is an efficient heat transfer mechanism. But blood is also needed in the organs and muscles to deliver oxygen and nutrients. Hot weather requires the circulatory system to do two conflicting jobs, especially if physical activity is increasing the demand for the blood to deliver oxygen and nutrients to working muscles.

Once blood moves heat to the skin, the heat can be lost in four ways: radiation, convection, conduction, and evaporation of sweat. But the first three mechanisms only work if the skin is warmer than its surroundings. On a hot, sunny day, the body will gain heat by radiation. Only a cool wind will carry heat away by convection, and conduction removes heat only if the body is in contact with something cooler. When air temperature is as high as skin temperature (normally no more than 93° F), **evaporation of sweat** is the only way that the body can lose heat. But after losing 3% to 5% of its water (1 or 2 liters) from sweating, which depletes blood volume, the body stops shunting extra blood to the skin because circulation to vital organs is more critical. Sweating then does little good, because most of the body's heat is no longer getting to the skin.

Water and salt

If you drink only when you are thirsty, you can get **dehydrated**. An **acclimatized** person who is working hard in warm surroundings can sweat up to 3 liters per hour. In one experiment with volunteers in the military, they did strenuous exercise in hot weather. Water was available but on average they did not drink until they had lost 2 liters, and when they drank they replaced only two-thirds of the water they had lost (**voluntary dehydration**).

Even if you are not acclimatized, you can sweat a liter or more per hour in hot weather. You will also be losing water through your breath in dry air and from urination.

Usually, about half a liter is as much as you can comfortably drink at once. Also, it takes time for water to pass out of the stomach (**gastric emptying**) and be absorbed by the intestine. In an average adult, about 1.2 liters of water per hour can be absorbed, and 3 liters per hour is as much as the stomach can tolerate (the gastric nausea threshold). This makes it hard to catch up with water loss after becoming dehydrated. So you should begin drinking water before you start exercising in the heat. Coffee and regular tea should be avoided because the caffeine in them is a **diuretic**. It increases water loss through urination. Alcohol also dehydrates by increasing urination.

Sweat and urine contain sodium and potassium. These are **electrolytes** that control the movement of water in and out of the body's cells. Some cases of water intoxication, also called **hyponatremia** ("too little salt") have been reported in Grand Canyon hikers and marathon runners, who were forcing themselves to drink a lot of water. But they were all either not eating anything or eating only sweets. When you're both losing and drinking a lot of water, you need to maintain your electrolyte balance with salty snacks such as trail mix of potassium-rich nuts and dried fruit, or with electrolyte drink.

You can make your own electrolyte mixture to add to your water. For each liter, mix 1/2 teaspoon salt (sodium chloride), 1/2 teaspoon baking soda (sodium bicarbonate), 1/4 teaspoon salt substitute (potassium chloride), and sugar or honey to taste. Alternate this drink with equal amounts of plain water.

Cool heads: Dressing for the heat

The brain has its own cooling system using blood vessels that pass through the skull to connect with circulation in the face. Blood picks up heat from the brain and carries it to the skin where it can be dissipated. Wearing a hat with a brim helps cool the head by shading the face, and a bandanna hanging from the back of the hat can shade the neck. Keeping the hat wet also cools the head by evaporation. A more high-tech solution is a fan built into the hat in front, powered by a solar battery on top.

Loose clothing lets air circulate around the skin, cooling by convection. Cotton absorbs up to 100% of its weight in water, and then becomes a vapor barrier, preventing your sweat from evaporating through the fabric. So it is not a good choice for vigorous activity in hot (or cold) weather. Most sports clothing for vigorous activity is made of synthetic fabrics such as polyester knit, which absorbs only 1% to 2% of its weight in water and dries quickly. So sweat evaporates through the pores (along with your excess heat) instead of saturating the fabric.

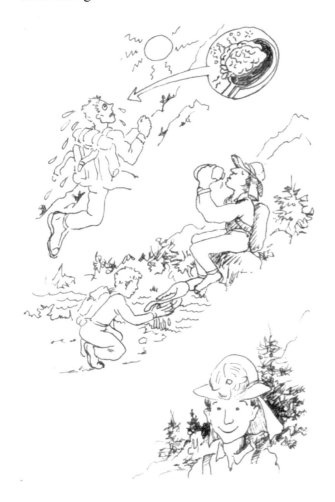

The climber at the top is overheating and getting dehydrated. At the stream, one hiker is hydrating and the other is wetting his hat to cool his head by evaporation. The bottom hiker has a solar-powered fan in his hat.

Heat production and heat loss

How much heat does your body produce, and how much can your sweat dissipate? At rest, a man of average size might produce about 60 kilocalories (kcal) of heat per hour. On a hot day, a seminude person at rest could gain up to 250 more kcal per hour from exposure to the sun, and a clothed person up to 100 kcal per hour (**solar load**). One kcal will heat one liter of water 1° C (2.2° F). During vigorous and sustained exercise, heat production can be multiplied up to 6 times in a fit person, and up to 10 times in an athlete. If heat production is multiplied 6 times, then an average sized man will be producing 360 kcal of heat per hour. If we assume that the man has 40 liters of water in his body, disregarding the solids, the heat will raise the temperature of the water by 9° C (16.2° F). That would be more than enough heat to broil the victim slowly in his own fluids, though he would have collapsed long before driving his body temperature so high.

Evaporating one liter of sweat from the skin will take away about 580 Kilocalories of heat. But first the circulatory system needs to carry the heat from the organs and working muscles that produce it to the skin, as well as supplying the sweat glands with water. Blood vessels under the skin can increase their blood flow 10 times. If you are dehydrated, however, your blood volume will be reduced. The circulatory system may not be able to spare enough blood from the vital organs to move heat to the skin or to deliver enough water to replenish the sweat glands.

Sweat can only take heat away from the skin if it evaporates. Clothing that absorbs sweat also prevents it from dissipating heat by evaporating. In dry air, sweat evaporates insensibly. But water vapor in the air (**humidity**) exerts vapor pressure, which inhibits evaporation of sweat. At 70% relative humidity (70% of maximum water vapor saturation in the air), sweat. just pools and drips off the skin, not cooling the body. The more humid the air, the lower the temperature at which heat risk begins. So heat loss by evaporation of sweat seldom reaches its optimum level because of all the limiting factors. Reduce heat risk by getting out of the heat when you are resting, to ease the stress on the circulatory system.

Heat risk factors

Risk factors for heat illness include being obese, fatigued, out of condition, or un-acclimatized to heat. Prior heat illness or recent fever may also handicap response to heat. Cardiovascular illness and diabetes weaken the circulatory system, and thus reduce its ability to cope with heat. Malaria (prickly heat) or healed burns impair sweating. Some drugs increase the risk of heat illness. Diuretics ("flowing through") including alcohol and caffeine increase fluid loss through urination, and blood volume is reduced with dehydration. Heat production is increased by amphetamines, cocaine, and some antidepressants. Antihistamines and some medications prescribed for psychiatric problems reduce sweating.

Heat illness

Even standing in the heat can cause fainting (**heat syncope**), because blood is drawn to the skin and pools in the legs, reducing blood pressure and cardiac output. A sodium deficiency in exercising muscles can cause **heat cramps**. Heat cramps are usually relieved by an electrolyte drink. It also helps to stretch out the cramping muscle.

Exercising in the heat can cause dehydration and collapse (**heat exhaustion**) if it overloads the circulatory system. In heat exhaustion, the body core temperature may be normal or a few degrees high. The patient will usually be sweating profusely. Severe dehydration can reduce blood volume, which will make the pulse rapid and weak. Symptoms of heat exhaustion may include headache, faintness, confusion, and nausea, all related to poor blood supply in vital organs from a stressed circulatory system. Treatment is to move the patient out of the heat and gradually rehydrate, adding electrolytes if plain water doesn't improve the patient's condition. If there is no shade, placing wet cloths on the head and neck can help prevent the patient from overheating.

If the body core temperature goes up past about 106° F (41° C), the temperature control system fails (heat stroke). **Classic heat stroke** (CHS), the slow cooker, may take days to develop. It usually afflicts the elderly unable to get out of the heat. However, even healthy athletes can generate enough heat from exercise to go into **exertional heat stroke** or EHS (the fast cooker) in as little as 15 minutes. More often than not, EHS victims will still be sweating profusely, with a rapid and bounding pulse. So the appearance of the skin is not a reliable way to distinguish heat stroke from heat exhaustion. Also, taking a rectal temperature in the field is seldom practical.

Behavior changes drastically in EHS, and is a more reliable way to distinguish it from heat exhaustion. Patients often become irrational, and sometimes aggressive. They may also have seizures, and if not cooled, go into a coma. The longer coma lasts, the less chance of survival. When in doubt, cool the patient.

Cooling

Cool water baths at 59° F (15° C) are just as effective as ice baths if the water is stirred to prevent a warm layer from forming around the body. Monitor vital signs, including level of responsiveness (by talking to the patient), and be careful not to over-cool. Misting (aerosols driven by fans) is used on pilgrims to Mecca. The water droplets act as artificial sweat, cooling the patient by evaporating from the skin. However, this method may not be so effective in a climate where humidity is high. Ice bags in towels against the big veins in the groin, armpit, and the sides of the neck, plus fanning and sponging, will also cool though not nearly as fast as immersion. Do not, however, use alcohol for cooling the skin. It can be absorbed into the blood causing alcohol intoxication.

Acclimatizing

Endurance training helps prepare you for heat stress, because even in cool weather, sustained aerobic exercise can generate enough heat to raise the body core temperature and stimulate some acclimatization. However, full acclimatization requires exercise in a warm environment. The body adapts to repeated heat stress in two ways. First, it becomes more efficient so that the metabolic cost of work and the heat produced by it are lower. Second, it improves heat loss mechanisms.

With aerobic conditioning, the heart pumps more blood with each stroke, so that it needs fewer contractions to move the same amount of blood. Sweating starts earlier when you are aerobically conditioned or acclimatized; and the maximum amount of sweat per hour increases. Also, the sweat glands and kidneys conserve sodium, losing only a tenth as much in sweat and urine. If your sweat no longer stings your eyes and tastes bland, you are either in good aerobic condition or at least partly acclimatized. A few days of acclimatizing will improve performance in heat. But the process continues for months, so those who live in a hot climate have an advantage over those exposed at short notice.

Cold

If you are losing heat faster than you can produce it, then your body temperature will drop. This is called **hypothermia** (Greek *hypo* "under" *thermia* "heat"). Vital organs, especially the brain, get less efficient when chilled. For this reason, hypothermia has probably caused many more accidents and deaths in the wilderness than accident statistics suggest.

Size and shape

Heat loss depends on the surface area of the skin, which increases roughly as the square of the height. Heat production depends on the volume of lean body tissue, which increases as the cube of height. Big people, therefore, have an advantage over small people in cold weather, because their ratio of heat-producing tissue to skin area is higher. For example, a 3-foot child will generally lose heat at least twice as fast as a 6-foot adult; a 1-foot tall infant at least 4 times as fast. Smaller people also transfer heat faster by conduction from the core to the skin, because their organs and muscles are closer to the surface.

Elderly people tend to have less lean muscle mass to produce heat and weak circulatory systems. As a result, their body temperatures may be below average even before exposure. They are more likely to have chronic diseases, or take medications that can interfere with heat production or temperature regulation. They also may not sense the cold as well as younger people and often fail to shiver.

Hypothermia and the brain

Chilling progressively affects all brain functions, including temperature regulation. Below 95° F brain temperature, memory and concentration are impaired, thinking slows down, and auditory or visual hallucinations are possible. **Speech** becomes slurred and increasingly difficult. Fine **coordination**

(especially of the fingers) deteriorates. Hypothermic patients often lose emotional expression (flat affect). Even mild hypothermia can bring out and exaggerate pre-existing behavioral problems, such as anxiety, poor judgment, or psychosis (living in a separate reality).

As the core temperature falls below 90° F, reflexes get more and more sluggish. **Muscle strength** also declines. Usually the knee jerk reflex is the last to go and the first to come back with rewarming. Voluntary movements are slowed, and the patient has serious problems with coordination and **balance**. A patient who is still conscious at an 86° F core temperature may take 15-30 seconds to touch the nose. **Pupils** become dilated and eye movement may be uncoordinated (i.e., the patient becomes cross-eyed). In an unresponsive hypothermic, pupil response to light will be so slow that you may miss it.

Breathing and circulation

Metabolism in cold tissues, including muscles, is less efficient. With a 1.1° F drop in body core temperature it takes half again as much oxygen to do the same amount of work. Because blood vessels in the limbs constrict to conserve heat (peripheral vasoconstriction), muscles and nerves in the limbs get less circulation and chill even more rapidly than the body core. As body temperature drops below 90° F, carbon dioxide (CO_2) in blood no longer increases breathing, so **breathing** slows. Mucus secretion increases and may clog air passages. The patient may become nauseated, so you need to be alert to prevent the aspiration of vomit.

The **pulse** soon slows down, sometimes to one-half of its normal rate, because the chilled heart pumps more slowly. It also pumps less with each stroke, so a hypothermic patient's pulse is hard to find, especially in the limbs, where circulation is reduced by peripheral vasoconstriction. If the pulse remains rapid, then something else is going on (e.g., drug overdose, hypoglycemia, or hypovolemic shock).

Another problem that can occur in deep hypothermia is **embolism** or blood clots because cold and thickened blood clots more easily. Water moves from blood to the tissues and can reduce blood volume as much as 25%. Cold suppresses the thirst sensation, so **dehydration** from increased urination and the failure to drink water can further reduce blood volume.

Digestion and metabolism

Heat production is increased by cold stress as long as the cells have enough fuel, water, and oxygen and body temperature remains normal. At lower blood temperatures, however, it is harder for glucose to cross cell membranes, less insulin is released by the pancreas, and cells become insulin resistant. Glucose may then accumulate in the blood (**hyperglycemia**) or be excreted in urine. Also, chilled kidneys cannot concentrate urine, so increased urination dehydrates the body. This is called **cold weather diuresis** ("flowing through"). Urine-soaked clothing is common in cases of profound hypothermia.

Metabolism slows down, so the body produces less heat. Below about 90° F, the gastrointestinal system stops functioning, which means that no new fuel goes into the blood from food. There will be no bowel sounds, and the abdominal muscles may be rigid. You should still, however, try to rule out injuries or illnesses that can also cause guarding or rigidity of the abdomen, in case their signs are masked by hypothermia.

Alcohol impairs judgment and concentration, and gives an illusory sense of warmth by dilating blood vessels near the skin, which suppresses shivering and may increase heat loss. Alcohol also seems to reduce heat production; and it can double urinary output, which is already increased by exposure to cold, thus dehydrating the patient much more rapidly.

Carbon monoxide from cooking in a tent increases hypothermia risk, because it reduces the oxygen-carrying capacity of the blood.

Treatment

Patients who are still alert, shivering, and coordinated should be able to restore their own body temperatures to normal if their heat loss is reduced by shelter and warm, dry clothing. Also, their heat production can be increased by re-hydration and energy food. Even patients who are confused and uncoordinated may respond to passive rewarming, if they are in a warm environment. In the field, however, when rapid evacuation is not possible, you may need to add heat.

Heat packs or hot water bottles (carefully wrapped to prevent burning) can warm blood going to the brain and other vital organs, if placed against the sides of the neck and in the armpits. Skin to skin warming should only be to the upper body, and the sleeping bag should be pre-warmed before putting the patient in it. Never massage a hypothermic. Warming the skin can suppress shivering, and stimulating circulation in the limbs would return cold, acidotic blood to the heart.

Handle hypothermics gently, especially if they are stiff and unresponsive. Heart tissue becomes very irritable when chilled, so jarring or rough handling, as well as exertion, can trigger ventricular fibrillation - a condition in which the heart muscle fibers twitch irregularly so that the heart does not pump blood.

A stiff and unresponsive hypothermic patient cannot be rewarmed with the resources you will have in the wilderness. The most you can achieve is to reduce or prevent further heat loss with a hypothermia wrap and arrange for an evacuation:

- Carefully strip off wet clothes (or cut them off if necessary to avoid jostling the patient).
- Dress the patient in dry clothes.
- Lay several foam pads and a pre-warmed sleeping bag on a tarp.
- Gently slide the patient into a sleeping bag.
- Wrap the tarp around the bag.

CPR on hypothermic patients is rarely successful without rapid transport to a hospital equipped for rewarming as well as advanced life support. In addition to ventricular fibrillation and embolisms, rewarming complications may include pneumonia from aspiration of mucus or vomit, and damage to the pancreas.

Immersion hypothermia

In cold water, we lose heat much faster than in air, because water conducts heat 25 times as fast as air and has a huge heat capacity. Body shape and composition, however, make much more difference in water than in cold air. Seals, walruses, and whales are insulated with a thick layer of blubber. At 48° F water temperature, an unprotected lean survivor will lose heat about 100 times as fast as in equally cold air, and up to 9 times as fast as a fat survivor in water. **Protective clothing** (a wet suit or dry suit) will reduce heat loss considerably. Personal flotation devices (PFD) also help keep you warmer in water, because they have a layer of insulating foam and keep your head out of the water. If you are wearing a PFD, you can conserve heat by doubling up and grasping your knees, or huddling with other survivors; but getting even part of your body out of the cold water by climbing onto floating wreckage is more efficient.

Immersion in water colder than about 60° F causes **changes in breathing**, as the body reacts to the sudden loss of heat. First, there is usually a reflex gasp, which may cause you to aspirate water. Then for several minutes, hyperventilation (up to five times normal) flushes out CO_2. Hyperventilation can cause confusion and muscle rigidity, and it decreases underwater breath-holding time (from 60 to 20 seconds in one experiment). This means less chance of survival in rough water or of escape from a submerged vehicle.

However, after the first few minutes of immersion, breathing slows to a rate and volume just sufficient to maintain metabolism. Systolic **blood pressure** rises. **Pulse rate** will increase for a few minutes, then slow down. Blood vessels near the surface dilate, probably because their muscular sheaths are paralyzed by cold, which may increase the rate of heat loss.

All of your muscles will get weaker and less efficient as they are chilled, so you may not be able to swim more than 15 minutes without protection in cold water. Even wearing a PFD, the average person can swim only about half a mile in 50°F water. Soon you may not have enough strength left to grip anything or climb out of the water.

Victims of immersion hypothermia should be pulled out of the water horizontally if possible and never be allowed to get up and walk. Blood pressure usually drops when someone emerges from cold water, and the effect is aggravated by standing and walking. Some reports tell of shipwreck survivors who were able to climb out of the water, then collapsed and died.

Submersion and drowning

Reactions to immersion in cold water increase the risk of drowning: loss of decision making ability as the brain is chilled; weakening of chilled muscles; and aspiration of water from the reflex gasp. Aspirating even a small amount of water can cause a laryngospasm – a reflexive constriction of the larynx – that normally keeps water out of the lungs, but also prevents breathing. If the laryngospasm does not release until the victim becomes unconscious, then (without a PFD) that victim will usually aspirate water and sink, because buoyancy depends on the amount of air in the lungs, as well as body fat and clothing.

Aspirated water can also have delayed effects on a drowning victim who has been revived, especially if the water was polluted. So any drowning victim who survived the experience should be evacuated - even one who seems fully recovered.

The classic mantra for water rescue is: reach; throw; row; go. Reach from land with something the victim can grab if possible. Throw a rope or floatation device to a victim too far to reach. If that is not possible, approach the victim in a boat. Swimming to the victim is the last resort, and should only be attempted by those trained in water rescue. If you are caught in swift water, try to turn on your back with your feet downstream so that your legs (and not your head) can absorb the impact of any collisions.

Once the patient is out of the water, check the airway, give oxygen if available, and do CPR if necessary. About 86% of drowning victims vomit during CPR (usually from swallowed water); so you must be prepared to turn the victim quickly onto the left side and clear vomitus from the mouth and nose. Victims of warm water submersion who do not revive after 30 minutes of resuscitation are usually considered dead; but victims of cold water drowning have been revived after 60 minutes of submersion, so the same principle applies to them as to victims of hypothermia by exposure: not dead until warmed and dead.

Frostbite & Raynaud's disease

In cold surroundings, heat from underlying tissues warms the skin, so skin must be cooled below 25° F in order to freeze. As the skin cools, blood flow to it decreases, dropping to a tenth of normal in the hands and feet at 59° F. But skin temperatures below 59° F trigger a protective reaction called cold-induced vasodilation (CIVD), also called hunter's response. Blood vessels dilate at short intervals to bring surges of warm blood to the skin. People who grow up and work in cold climates, such as Inuit, Lapps, and Nordic fishermen tend to have strong CIVDs.

If the body core temperature is dropping, however, or temperature in the exposed tissues drops to the 37°-50° F range, circulation withdraws from the surface and the extremities, because the vital organs have higher priority. Then temperature in the extremities can drop as rapidly as 1° F per minute.

Raynaud's disease

Some people have a negative circulatory response to cold – Raynaud's disease. Their circulatory systems withdraw blood from the extremities in cold weather even when the air temperature is well above freezing, which means that their hands and feet can easily go numb. In sub-freezing weather, they have no natural defenses against frostbite.

Any sudden drop in skin temperature can trigger Raynaud's disease in a susceptible person. Hands or feet turn pale as blood withdraws, and the victim may also feel tingling and numbness. It can happen in mild as well as cold weather. Circulatory problems and some drugs can bring it on, but the mechanism of primary Raynaud's disease, caused by cold or stress, is unknown.

Murray P. Hamlet, who ran the U.S. Army's Cold Research Division, developed and tested a simple procedure for treating primary Raynaud's disease, which reconditions the circulatory system to increase blood flow in the hands and feet when the body is exposed to cold. He claims to have a high success rate. You need a warm place and a cold place, with a tub of water, kept at 110° F, in each place. Dress lightly.

In the warm room, immerse your hands in the hot water for two to five minutes. Then wrap your hands in a towel, go to the cold area, and immerse your hands for ten minutes. Repeat the cycle three to six times on alternate days, for a total of about 50 trials. The reconditioning usually lasts for years and can be quickly restored if it lapses.

Frostbite

We lose sensation at a skin temperature of about 50° F, so numb skin is not necessarily frozen. To test for actual freezing, dent the skin with your fingernail. If the skin remains dented like wax, it is frozen, but the frostbite is superficial. If the skin cannot be dented, then underlying tissues are also frozen. Some authorities recommend rewarming superficial frostbite in the field with body heat if you can't get indoors, but deep frostbite should never be deliberately thawed until the patient is in an environment that can be kept warm. Victims can walk on frozen feet, if necessary, but thawed frostbite is crippling as well as being very painful. Moreover, the damaged tissues quickly refreeze in sub-freezing weather.

Our extremities are most vulnerable to frostbite, because they are furthest from the heart, their tissues are close to the surface, and they have a high surface-to-volume ratio. This makes them efficient at radiating heat. Feet are frozen more often than hands, because feet also lose heat by conduction to cold ground, rock, or snow. Tight boots greatly increase the risk of frostbite because they impair circulation to the feet, which have little heat-producing tissue of their own and depend on a constant supply of warm blood to keep from freezing in very cold weather. Ears and noses are also vulnerable, and some winter joggers have suffered frostbitten scrotums and penises. Also, keeping unprotected eyes open against a cold wind can freeze the corneas, for example when snowmobiling or cross-country skiing.

Risk factors
- hypothermia (blood withdraws to vital organs);
- wind chill
- alcohol consumption (increases heat loss and lowers heat production);
- smoking (causes blood vessels to constrict);
- impaired circulation to hands or feet, e.g. from tight boots;
- immobility (e.g., when trapped by a storm);
- accident (physical and psychological effects);
- fatigue or apathy (slows heat production);
- previous frostbite injury (damaged blood vessels);
- wet skin cools faster than dry skin and can trigger ice crystallization in the tissues.

Contact with very cold metal can freeze skin instantly, especially a full metal fuel container. To prevent contact, wear glove liners, and cover metal (such as fuel bottles for backpacking stoves) with duct tape. Petroleum fuels can chill far below the freezing point of water and remain liquid, so they can also freeze skin on contact. Liquified petroleum fuels such as butane, which are pressurized natural gas, are even more dangerous. They can freeze skin on contact in any weather, as they suddenly expand from liquid to gas.

Treatment
Photos courtesy of Ben Schifrin, MD

If the skin is getting numb, it is close to the temperature at which circulation will withdraw, leaving the tissues defenseless against freezing. Outdoors, body heat may be the only way to rewarm the skin (putting your fingers into your armpits or inside the clothing, for example). Another technique is to force circulation back into the hands by shaking them vigorously or windmilling the arms. It is more difficult to rewarm your own feet, unless you are an advanced yogi. Sometimes the only alternative is to find a friend with a warm belly, as Thomas Hornbein did on his ascent of the west ridge of Mt. Everest. He came back with all his toes, but his companion (who did not rewarm his feet) lost all his toes to frostbite.

Portable handwarmers, which weigh only a few ounces, can deliver heat to a small area for hours. They may be the only way to prevent frostbite in a fractured limb, if evacuation is delayed. Even superficial frostbite is better rewarmed indoors, because if it refreezes after thawing, the damage will be worse and probably go deeper.

For deep frostbite, prevent further heat loss during evacuation with dry, loose wraps or clothing, and pad or splint for protection if the injury is to an extremity. Transport to a hospital or, if that is not possible, to another place where the patient can be kept warm. Thaw an extremity by immersing it in water at 104° to 108° F. Stir when adding new hot water. Have the patient move the thawing digits, if possible, but do not massage. Continue warming until the skin is red and pliable (up to 30 minutes).

After removing the thawed digits from the water, gently separate fingers or toes with loose, sterile dressings, elevate, and handle as little as possible. After rewarming, the goal of treatment is to maintain circulation in the thawed tissue while preventing infection. Swelling and blisters develop within hours.

Damage to blood vessels in the thawed tissues continues, probably caused by clots. Physicians no longer amputate, unless the limb dies from impaired circulation, or infection gets out of control. Nature does a slower but better job of separating living from dead tissue. Dead tissues blacken and wither over weeks or months. If damage is bone-deep, the dead part of the limb eventually self-amputates. If enough tissue survives to keep the limb viable, the blackened tissue will peel off, revealing new skin underneath.

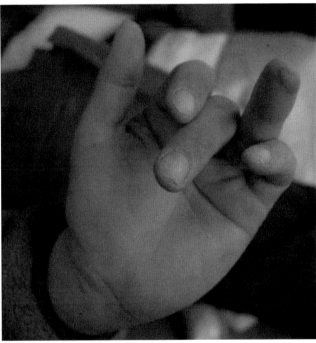

Frostbitten fingers at 21,000 feet

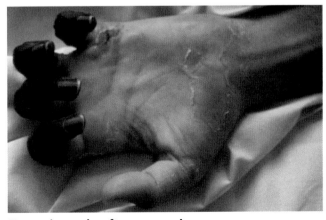

Necrosis weeks after rewarming

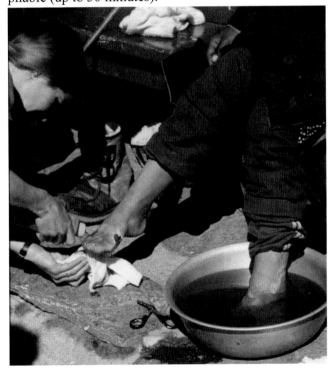

Rewarming frostbitten feet in warm water.

Effects of high altitude

Atmospheric air is about 21% oxygen. At 18,000 feet, atmospheric pressure is about one-half sea level pressure, and at the top of Mt. Everest (29,029 feet), about one-third of sea level pressure. Inhaling mixes fresh air with the oxygen-depleted residual air still in the lungs, which lowers the percentage of oxygen to as little as 13% in the alveoli. So partial pressure of oxygen decreases when it is inhaled from the atmosphere into the alveoli (air sacs) of the lungs. Inhaling and exhaling more deeply makes the mixture richer, reducing the drop in oxygen pressure from atmosphere to alveoli (below).

Oxygen is driven through the body by pressure differences, from higher to lower concentrations. From the alveoli, it moves across the membranes and thin capillary walls into the blood, which carries oxygen through the pulmonary veins to the left side of the heart. The left ventricle then pumps the oxygenated blood through the aorta to the whole body.

Hemoglobin in red blood cells bonds to oxygen where oxygen pressure is high (in capillaries around the alveoli) and releases oxygen from capillaries to the working cells, where oxygen pressure is low. Iron in hemoglobin gives blood cells their color: bright red when it binds to oxygen, and darker red when the oxygen is released.

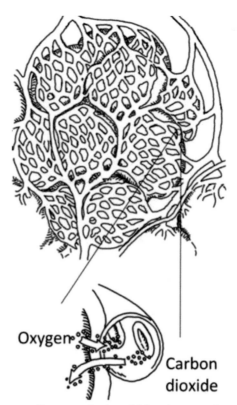

Oxygen depleted blood, returning to the right side of the heart, is pumped to the lungs by the right ventricle through the pulmonary arteries. This blood also carries dissolved carbon dioxide (CO_2), a waste product of metabolism, and some of it is expelled as you exhale.

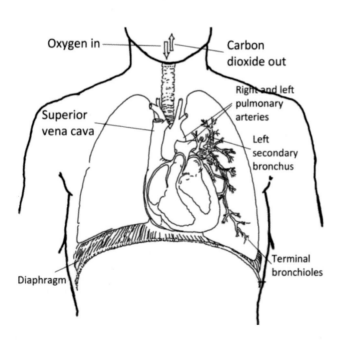

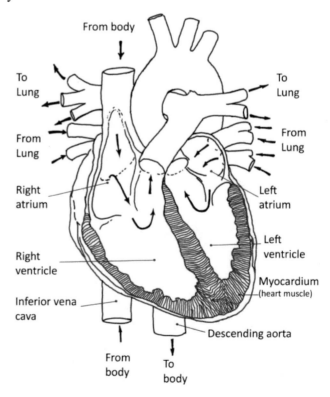

Breathing and altitude

Carbon dioxide, dissolved in blood, forms a weak acid. As it accumulates, it makes the blood more acidotic, which stimulates the respiratory center in the brain to increase breathing. As we flush carbon dioxide out of the lungs by breathing more rapidly or deeply, however, the blood becomes more alkaline, which decreases breathing. Two sensors in the carotid arteries of the neck also signal the respiratory center to increase breathing as oxygen concentration decreases

Up to about 5,000 feet, oxygen saturation in hemoglobin remains about as high as at sea level - at least 96%. As we go higher, breathing must become both deeper and more regular to compensate for thinner air. The body dumps bicarbonates from the blood through the urine, which allows a lower concentration of carbon dioxide to make the blood acidotic, and to stimulate the breathing center of the brain. This is the most important way that the body acclimatizes to high altitude.

At high altitude, the heart has less blood to pump, because of dehydration and a shift of fluid out of the circulatory system. To compensate and meet oxygen demand, the heart rate increases (up to 50% at 19,000 to 25,000 feet). Blood pressure also increases slightly, but usually returns to normal in a few days (except in the pulmonary arteries) as climbers acclimatize to altitude. Heart rate decreases with acclimatization, but remains above sea-level values. Above 5,000 feet, even acclimatized people lose about 3% of their work capacity for every 1,000 feet of elevation gain. So at the top of Mt. Everest a climber's work capacity would be only about one-quarter what it was at sea level.

Helping the body to Acclimatize

Although the physiology of the body at high altitude is complex, the ways in which we can help our bodies to acclimatize are simple:
- Gain altitude gradually.
- Drive to the high trailhead the night before starting the climb and sleep there to start acclimatizing.
- Climb high, and sleep lower.
- Drink water regularly. Dehydration dries up the urine supply and prevents the body from dumping bicarbonates.
- Stay warm. Muscles become much less efficient as they chill.
- Avoid respiratory depressants such as alcohol and sleeping pills.
- Don't climb high with a respiratory infection. Colds and flu set you up for altitude illness.

Other responses to altitude

Hemoglobin production starts within two hours of ascent, and new red blood cells are in circulation within four to five days. Total body water decreases at high altitude because of losses through urination, sweating, and breathing. Loss of the thirst sensation and the difficulty of melting snow reduce the chances that lost water will be replaced. Blood volume is reduced because water that the circulatory system delivers to the sweat glands and various parts of the body is not fully replaced. More red blood cells make the blood even thicker, which slows circulation and increases the risk of blood clots.

Because altitude exposure reduces mental and physical efficiency, it increases the risk of accidents. Another problem is that wounds heal more slowly with altitude gain, especially in the extremities, because too little oxygen is reaching the tissues. The effects of altitude form a spectrum or continuum. Patients often progress from a mild to a more serious condition. But for convenience, altitude illness is classified into several clinical types.

Acute Mountain Sickness (AMS)

Acute Mountain Sickness may begin with ascent above 6,000 feet, but is more common 6 to 48 hours later. Symptoms vary, but headache (often intense) is the most common. It is usually not relieved by aspirin, though ibuprofen may help. Other symptoms may include weakness, lassitude, shortness of breath, nausea, loss of appetite, and insomnia. AMS often interferes with sleep, and sleep loss can aggravate the effects of altitude.

Even though most AMS victims are probably dehydrated as well as being short of oxygen, fluid leaking out of the blood vessels water-logs the tissues in the brain, lungs, and digestive system. Diuresis (increased urination, encouraged by drinking plenty of water) makes climbers less susceptible to altitude illness. In the face and limbs, edema can be uncomfortable, but it is not dangerous unless it affects the lungs or the brain.

Treatment of AMS is to stop ascending until the body catches up with the altitude, rehydrate, and watch for improvement or worsening of the condition. If the symptoms persist, go down. Often just going down 1,000 feet or so will enable you to sleep, recover, and then continue the ascent.

Acetazolamide (Diamox) may relieve or prevent AMS. Acetazolamide speeds up the process of dumping bicarbonates from the blood. This increases the effective level of carbon dioxide in the blood and thus tends to make breathing deeper and more regular, especially while sleeping. Since it does this by increasing urination, it is especially important to stay hydrated when taking acetazolamide. But people who are allergic to sulfa drugs cannot take acetazolamide. A natural remedy, Ginkgo biloba (which dilates blood vessels and thus lowers blood pressure) has also been shown to help prevent AMS and reduce its severity.

High Altitude Pulmonary Edema (HAPE)

If parts of the lung are poorly ventilated (hypoxic), the pulmonary arteries supplying them constrict, directing more circulation to the rest of the lung. But at high altitude, the whole lung is hypoxic, so the response increases pulmonary arterial pressure (PAP), and may start leaking fluid into the alveoli. In x-rays, the accumulations of fluid (edema) look like fluffy snowballs scattered through the lung.

A climber getting High Altitude Pulmonary Edema (HAPE) will be short of breath and tired, even after resting, because the edema is reducing oxygen transfer in the lungs. Resting pulse rate will probably be over 100 per minute (or at least 30 more than what is normal for that patient), in response to low oxygen delivery. This speeding up of the resting pulse is perhaps the most reliable way to distinguish HAPE in its early stages from AMS. A climber who has these symptoms after resting needs to go down immediately.

As HAPE progresses, the patient will be coughing, dryly at first, and the congestion will produce a breath sound, called crackles, like the sound of hairs being rubbed between your fingers. Crackles can be heard with a stethoscope, or by putting your ear against the patient's rib cage under the armpit. As more fluid accumulates, the sound may turn into gurgling, and coughing may bring up sputum that is tinged pink with red blood cells. Lying down may make it worse because fluid in the lungs will cover more surface and reduce oxygen exchange.

Oxygen will help, especially if given through a positive pressure mask, but it will not reverse the course of HAPE, which is 50% fatal if not treated. Immediate treatment is descent to lower altitude. The Gamow bag, a portable nylon tube pressurized by a foot pump, can simulate lower altitude while waiting for evacuation. After recovery, the patient should be monitored for respiratory infection.

High Altitude Cerebral Edema(HACE)

Shortage of oxygen stimulates increased cerebral blood flow, which stretches blood vessels. Then fluid accumulates in and around the cells, increasing brain volume. Since the brain is enclosed in the skull, it cannot expand, and pressure increases.

This oxygen shortage and swelling can have many effects on brain function, from confusion and irritability in a mild case to amnesia, hallucinations, or irrational behavior in an advanced case. But the effect on the balance center of the brain, called **ataxia**, is the most important warning sign of HACE (high altitude cerebral edema), and the easiest to test. The Greek word "ataxia" means "without order," but what the ataxic patient lacks is a normal sense of balance.

To test for ataxia, have the patient walk a straight line, heel against toe. Doing it easily rules out HACE. Swaying indicates a mild case, going off-line a moderate case, and falling a severe case. Another ataxia test is to have the patient stand within (but not touching) your circled arms for 30 seconds, with feet together, hands on shoulders, and eyes closed. A stable posture rules out HACE. Swaying indicates a mild to moderate case, and a patient who falls against your arms has a severe case.

Treatment is to descend immediately, because otherwise the patient will probably be in a coma within 12 hours, and die. Most patients with HACE also have HAPE. Pumping up pressure in a Gamow bag can simulate lower altitude during (or while waiting for) evacuation, and oxygen will help. However, a patient with HACE must always be evacuated. Fortunately, HACE is the least common form of altitude illness, and almost unknown below 11,000 feet.

Vision and altitude

Since the retina is very sensitive to oxygen level in the blood, altitude affects vision. Night vision starts getting dim at 4,000 feet, and at higher altitudes you may suffer night blindness. Much less common are temporary visual changes, such as blurred or double vision. flashing lights, or blindness. These problems usually stop after descent.

Using contact lenses at high altitude is problematic. They reduce the oxygen supply to the cornea if left in overnight, but can be hard to keep clean in a wilderness environment if they are frequently removed and replaced. Also, they may freeze in their containers at night. Guidelines for military personnel include some sensible suggestions: use disposable lenses for up to 1 week; carry eye drops and contact lens re-wetting solution; and always carry back-up glasses, including prescription sunglasses or goggles that will fit over regular glasses.

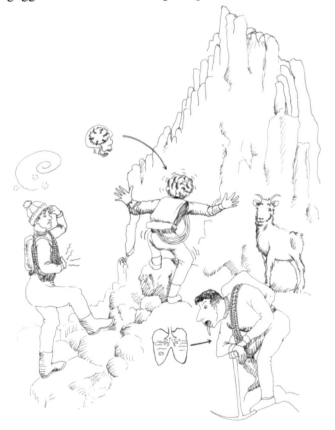

The climber on the left is feeling the typical headache and malaise of AMS. The climber in the center is losing his sense of balance because of HACE. The lungs of the climber on the right are filling with fluid (HAPE). The mountain goat, however, is having no problems with the altitude.

Other altitude Problems

Altitude can cause other problems as well, some of them serious. Clots in the thickened blood can break loose and be carried through the heart to the lungs (pulmonary embolism) or brain (stroke). Perhaps the most notorious altitude problem is HAFE (High-Altitude Flatus Expulsion). Because atmospheric pressure is lower, gasses inside the gut expand. HAFE is only dangerous, however, to the noses of other people in the tent.

Solar radiation

Ultraviolet (UVR) is the most dangerous solar radiation that penetrates the atmosphere, because it has the shortest wavelength, and therefore the highest energy, so too much exposure to UVR can damage skin, increasing the risk of skin cancer, as well as damaging unprotected eyes. The higher you climb, the greater the UVR exposure, with an increase of 8%-10% for every 1000 ft. of altitude gained. UVR exposure is also increased if you are on a reflecting surface. Clouds do not block UV, so it is easy to burn on an overcast day because you don't feel the need of sun protection.

In the United States, one person in five born today will get skin cancer; in Australia and New Zealand (because of the hole in the ozone layer), one out of three. Sun damage also ages skin prematurely, causing it to wrinkle and lose its elasticity. So you need to know how to protect your skin.

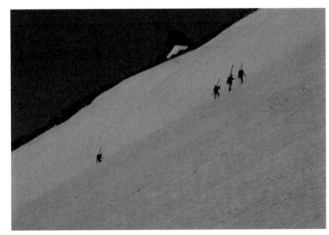

High altitude and a reflective surface both increase UV exposure.

Sunscreens and sun protection

Sunscreens help to prevent skin damage by absorbing the energy of ultraviolet radiation. Sun blocks (also called physical sunscreens) form a layer over the skin that reflects ultraviolet. Sunscreen labels have numbers that supposedly tell you how effective a sunscreen is – SPF (sun protection factor). If you multiply this SPF number by the time your unprotected skin could be exposed to sunlight without burning, you get the length of time that the manufacturer claims the sunscreen will protect you. The non-profit Environmental Working Group (http://www.ewg.org/2015sunscreen/) has a useful guide to sunscreens:

In response to UV exposure, your skin produces melanin, which absorbs, reflects, and scatters UV. As melanin oxidizes, it darkens the skin (tanning), though the skin may already be sunburned by the time that new melanin gets to it. People with more melanin-producing cells have darker skin and more natural sun protection.

You should apply sunscreen an hour before sun exposure, so that the active ingredient can bond to the outer layer of skin. Insect repellent applied over sunscreen will reduce its effectiveness by at least one third, because the repellent is in a solvent that will also dissolve part of the sunscreen. So apply insect repellent after the sunscreen has had time to bond to the skin.

Wet skin burns faster than dry skin, and no sunscreens could accurately be called waterproof. So you will have to reapply sunscreen frequently to exposed skin when you are sweating in hot weather.

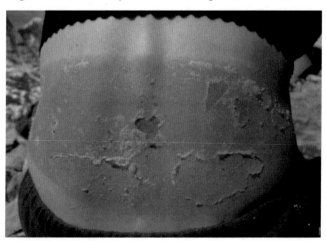

At 15,000 feet, it took only 15 minutes of exposure to cause this sunburn.

Sun blocks

Sun blocks (physical sunscreens) contain either zinc oxide or titanium dioxide particles that reflect UV, but to do this they need to stay on the skin. The ones with greasy bases are messy, but more tenacious. If the particles are ground very fine (micronized) the sun block is transparent to visible light, and does not have the classic clown-white effect.

Clothing

An alternative to sunscreens is protective clothing. A hat with a wide brim will help to protect the face, especially from the mid-day sun. Pinning a bandana to the back will protect the back of the neck. For extreme conditions (e.g., spring skiing at high altitude) consider wearing a hood of lightweight cloth with eye, nostril and mouth holes that hang over a hat. Mold the eyeholes around your sunglasses to maintain your field of vision.

Some clothing fabrics are tested for UV protection and given a UV protection factor (UPF) similar to the SPF for sunscreens. Tightness of weave and the material of the fabric are the most important factors. Some materials (like 100% polyester) absorb as well as block UV radiation, and others may have UV absorbers added to the fabric. Also, most wet fabrics transmit more UV than dry. For example, a dry white cotton T-shirt has a UPF of 5 or more, but it loses most of its protection when it is drenched with sweat.

Photosensitivity and allergic reactions

Many medications can cause photosensitivity in some people: antidepressants, antipsychotics, antihistamines, antimicrobials, diuretics, hypoglycemics, nonsteroidal anti-inflammatory drugs, and (ironically) sunscreens containing benzophenones or cinnamates. This results in exaggerated sunburn, out of proportion to exposure. Those with very fair skin who burn easily are most susceptible. At least 10% of Caucasians can get another reaction if exposed to more sunlight than usual - sun poisoning or polymorphous light eruption - especially at the first exposure of the season. As the name suggests, the reaction can take many forms, including swelling, blistering, and scabbing.

Vitamin C

Dr. Sheldon Pinnell, Chief of Dermatology at Duke University School of Medicine, showed in 1991 that vitamin C could reduce skin damage from UV if applied directly to the skin. It is not a sunscreen and does not replace sunscreen, but it will reduce the amount of damage done by the UV that penetrates the screen. Just dissolve vitamin C crystals in water and rub the solution on your skin before going out into the sun. The solution will be absorbed by the skin in concentrations 20 times as great as you can achieve by eating the vitamin. When rubbed on and absorbed by the skin, vitamin C has a half-life of 10-20 days, which means that at the end of that time half of what you originally applied will be left.

Sunglasses and ultraviolet radiation

Ultraviolet filtering or absorption depends on the lens material, thickness and the way it is processed. An absorptive tint may be processed into the lens either while it is being made or in the final stages while it is being ground to prescription. Most glass lenses are tinted during the early stages of production. This kind of tint is permanent, and its light transmission does not change over time. It also reduces internal reflection, because the tint is distributed throughout the lens. Plastic lenses are tinted by surface absorption, in which the tint solution penetrates 3-4 microns into the resin surface. This type of tint fades with time.

Photochromatic glass lenses, that darken when exposed to light, were introduced by Corning Glass Works in 1964. Silver and chloride ions are included in the glass melt, where they form silver halide microcrystals. When exposed to ultraviolet or blue light, these crystals dissociate into silver ions, which cluster into specks, absorbing all UVB, most UVA, and some visible light. In darker conditions, the specks split into atoms which form crystals again, transmitting more light. This process is reversible indefinitely and works without deterioration as long as the lenses last.

Photochromatic lenses darken as it gets cooler, and lighten as it gets warmer. Blocking of UV, however, is not affected by temperature. These lenses protect the eyes from harmful light, both visible and invisible in both dark and light conditions. Photochromatic or variable tint lenses called Transitions are available in plastic and polycarbonate. They are 50% lighter than glass and block 100% of the UV rays.

Image distortion in sunglasses can cause eyestrain and headaches. It is also dangerous in activities that require accurate vision. A good test for distortion (in a non-prescription lens) is to hold the lens in front of a movie or slide projector. If the image is unchanged, then the lens has good optical clarity. Alternatively, hold the lens at arm's length and look for any bending of a straight line, such as a doorway or window frame. Another test is to hold the lens up to a fluorescent light and rotate it. If the fluorescent tubes appear to change shape, the lenses do not have consistent optical clarity.

For every serious wilderness trip, the group should have at least one pair of extra sunglasses. Plastic lenses and nylon frames are the toughest and most likely to survive accidents. A hat with a visor shades the eyes. Sun shades can be cut out of cardboard or heavy paper in the shape of glasses, with a pinhole in the center of each cardboard lens. These will protect your eyes from UV and enable you to see short distances, but they will restrict your peripheral vision.

Lightning

Lightning can:

- strike directly if the victim is a prominent object in the area (about 5% of strikes);
- splash over from another prominent object such as an isolated tree (about 1/3 of strikes);
- flow through the ground from a nearby strike to shock the victim (about half of strikes);
- flow through a conductor such as water or a wire fence.

Current through the brainstem can damage the cardiorespiratory control centers, which would make resuscitation more difficult. This happens to about 75% of the victims in a direct strike, and about 67% in a splashover; but to only about 8% of victims injured by ground current, because typically most of the current goes up one leg and down the other. Victims of direct strike or splashover are also more likely to suffer temporary paralysis (two-thirds of them in the upper limbs only) or temporary blindness. Sometimes loss of vision can be permanent.

In about one-half of lightning strike victims, the concussion ruptures the eardrums, so the victim will not be able to hear you. Lightning can also cause trauma from muscle spasms, or from throwing the victim some distance. Burns are usually superficial, in a streaking pattern if the current flashing over the skin vaporizes sweat. Punctate burns may be caused by vaporized sweat droplets, or be exit wounds from current passing through deep tissues. Full thickness burns can be caused to skin in contact with synthetic clothing that the current melts. Flashover of current can also blast clothes off the body.

Treating the victims

A lightning strike victim may have secondary injuries from being hurled to the ground (like the man in the example above) or thrown through the air by the blast wave. But unless these injuries are severe enough to compromise the vital systems, there is a good chance of reviving the victim with prompt CPR. Even if the cardiorespiratory centers in the brain are damaged, and the victim does not resume breathing spontaneously, there is a good chance that the pulse will come back. In this case, continuing rescue breathing until the helicopter arrives can save a life. Rescue breathing is much easier to do than full CPR.

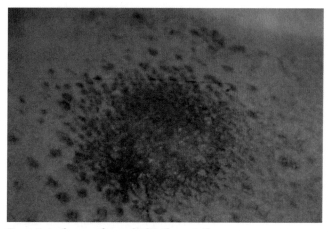

Punctate burns from lightning strike
Photo courtesy of Ben Schifrin, MD

Long-term effects

Fatality from lightning strike is about 30%. Only 100 to 300 deaths are reported each year in the United States. But survivors can suffer long-term neurological effects that are still poorly understood. One survivor, Gretel Ehrlich, has written a vivid account of her experience. She was struck twice, first by ground current flowing up the legs of her horse and bouncing a spark off her head, then years later by a direct hit.

When she woke up after the direct hit, her eye crusted with blood, she thought she was dead. Her heart was beating erratically, and she was partially paralyzed.

Although her wounds healed, she continued to have headaches, chest pains, and trouble staying conscious. Doctors denied her problems or were unable to help. Finally a cardiologist referred her to Joseph Ilvento, who specializes in the effects of electrical impulses (including lightning) on the heart. He found that damage to her brain stem prevented it from sending speedup signals to the heart in response to oxygen demand. Instead her heart slowed down, so she would often pass out when she stood up. Now she takes medications that maintain her heart rate and blood pressure.

Avoiding lightning strike

Since electricity follows the path of least resistance (POLR), high points in the landscape are likely targets for lightning. So the best way to avoid lightning strike is not to be a POLR and not to be on or near a POLR during thunderstorms. Clouds do not even have to be overhead for lightning to strike - many survivors report "blue sky" strikes.

In an open field or near a solitary tree, you are very exposed. Staying inside a forest is much safer. Failing that, huddling in a depression may reduce your exposure. Peaks and ridges are doubly dangerous, because lightning can blast you off them. Mountaineers have often reported tingling, humming through metal objects, and even St. Elmo's fire (a bluish glow or corona as the air is ionized). Sometimes they feel these sensations through their own bodies as static electricity builds up during a thunderstorm. These are urgent signals to get down to a less exposed place. If a group is caught in an exposed place, they should stay at least 20 feet apart because lightning can jump at least 15 feet (splashover) if it strikes one person.

Caves or overhangs are tempting, but unless a cave is deeper than it is wide, ground current from a nearby strike can flow over the surface. A group of hikers once learned this the hard way, when they continued their trip up Half Dome in Yosemite National Park in spite of storm warnings. When a thunderstorm caught them on top, they took shelter in a shallow cave near the edge. Ground current from a nearby lightning strike blew them out, and they fell to their deaths.

While the number of people struck by lightning is small, those who do outdoor activities are at the greatest risk, especially in the mountains, in open places, and on water. If you are caught in an exposed position, try to get to shelter or a place less exposed. If lightning does strike, and one or more people in your group are down, check the ones who are still and quiet first. If someone is not breathing, you have a good chance of saving a life by promptly giving rescue breaths and doing CPR if necessary.

Dressing for survival

Genetic engineers may someday enable us to grow winter coats of fur. Until then, however, we will need an artificial substitute – clothing – to survive in cold weather. Clothing, like fur, controls heat transfer by controlling the layer of air around the body. Air is an excellent insulator, so trapping it against the skin keeps heat in. Conversely, venting and circulating warmed air away from the skin carries heat away. And since our body's heat production can increase up to ten-fold when we are exercising hard, we often have to get rid of excess heat even in cool weather.

Water is an excellent conductor, and it can also absorb far more heat than air. If water displaces the trapped air around the skin, it will turn clothing into a refrigerator. Clothing therefore needs to control the movement of water as well as air. Keeping rainwater and snow out would be a simple function to design into clothing, if it did not also have to allow our sweat to evaporate into the air. Performing both these functions during active use requires clothing to have good design and the right materials.

The right stuff

Wool keeps sheep warm and dry, but the sheep have oil glands that keep the fibers water-repellent. We have only the oil that is left in the wool after manufacture. Wool garments can absorb up to half their weight in water, although they may not feel wet until they are 35% to 50% saturated. Also, wool dries very slowly. These limitations make wool best for clothing in which its toughness and resilience count: long-wearing socks, durable mittens, and tightly woven pants or shirts.

Cotton can quickly soak up 100% of its weight in water, and it loses 90% of its insulating value when wet, so it makes good bath towels but terrible cold-weather clothing. Down-filled garments are tempting because down's springy plumules expand more and trap more insulating air than any other material of the same weight. But down, like cotton, has high affinity for moisture and loses almost all of its insulating power when wet. Down clothing is, therefore, most useful in arctic conditions where it is unlikely to get wet, and where its warmth-to-weight ratio significantly lightens the burden of clothing.

Silk absorbs about 20% of its weight in water, so it makes a better inner layer than other natural fibers, and some people like the feel of it next to their skin. But it usually requires careful hand washing, and does not perform as well as synthetics.

Synthetic fibers have much more survival value than natural fibers in cold and wet weather, because they absorb very little water. Nylon can absorb only 4% of its weight in water, while polyester and polypropylene absorb 1% to 2%. If these fabrics get soaked, they feel clammy, but do not lose much insulating value. They dry out very fast, because the water does not wet the fibers in the fabric. In natural fabrics, by contrast, water bonds to the fibers, displacing trapped air bubbles. It requires a great deal of energy in the form of body heat to displace it.

Layering

Clothing for the body and limbs should be layered, so that it can easily be added or taken off to fit conditions and activity level. The inner layer should be stretchy, so that it hugs the body without binding, and should allow sweat to move freely between its fibers ("wicking off"). The middle layers are insulation, stabilizing the layer of air warmed by body heat next to the skin. They should also allow sweat to pass through. The outer layer, or shell, should keep wind and water out of the insulating warmed air. But like the other layers, it must allow evaporated sweat to escape. These conflicting functions make the shell the most difficult layer to design and sew, and often the most expensive.

The inner layer

Specially knit polyester comes in several thicknesses, from lightweight (for active use in moderate temperatures) to expedition weight (for severe cold). Polypropylene fishnet, however, is an excellent inner layer because it gives a lot of warmth for its weight.

The open mesh allows sweat to escape, which makes it comfortable over a large range of temperatures and activity levels. It is made by Brynjie (www.brynjie-shop.com), a Norwegian company.

Insulating layers

For active use, these should usually be of polyester pile or fleece. Its most common brand name is Polartec®. Fleece is synthetic fur with a short nap, inside and out. Wind-Pro® is more tightly knit Polartec®, which has about four times the wind resistance Pile is thick synthetic fur. Polyester is also used as fill, like down, for jackets that are sewn into compartments. These are good for staying warm when you're not moving, but not so good for active use because they do not vent sweat or excess heat. Also, they do not dry as easily as fleece or pile, because the compartments trap water.

Outer layer: Wind and rain Shell

Shells (parkas or anoraks, and rain pants) are of nylon or polyester, with a water-repellent layer laminated inside. To protect the water-repellent layer, they have either another layer of fabric laminated to the inside or a liner. They may also have a waxy coating sprayed or washed onto the outer layer that resists wetting.

If you do serious outdoor activities in extreme conditions, where your survival may depend on your clothing, then you need high quality outerwear. And if you spend much of the year outdoors, the comfort and safety margin of the best outerwear is still a good investment. But for occasional trips in moderate conditions, where you have an easy escape route, cheaper outerwear may be adequate. If you're huddling in the rain, or hiking on an easy trail, advanced design features aren't going to make much difference.

Head, hands and feet

Head protection: The hood of your parka should fit comfortably over your head insulation. A warm cap of synthetic or wool that pulls down over the ears, and a lightweight balaclava that can cover the whole head and neck, are a good combination. For very cold, windy conditions a neoprene facemask may be needed.

For the hands: Synthetic glove liners, gloves or mitts (wool or synthetic), and water-repellent overmitts are the three layers. The middle and outer layers may be combined into insulated gloves, but on a back-

country trip, these are hard to dry out when they get wet. Glove liners are essential so that you don't expose bare skin when you need full use of your fingers.

For the feet: Leather boots require preparation to make them waterproof. First, seal all seams, especially in the welt (connecting the uppers and the soles) with a liquid such as Stitch-Lock. This saturates the threads and makes them swell, sealing the stitch holes. Then seal the leather uppers by rubbing in a waterproofing compound for leather. Plastic ski and mountaineering boots are waterproof and insulated with foam. If they don't fit well, however, they can pinch and impair circulation. This problem in rented boots has caused more than one case of frostbite.

For cold winter skiing or mountaineering, gaiters should completely cover the boots and have pockets inside to insert insulating foam. Inside the boots, you need thin, synthetic inner socks that cling to the foot and protect the skin from abrasion. Thick wool or synthetic socks provide insulation, but be careful not to cram so many socks into the boots that you cut off circulation. To reduce heat loss by conduction through the bottom of the boot, add insoles of foam neoprene if they were not included with the boots.

Vapor barrier liners

Since we lose heat by insensible sweating, even in cold weather, some people use waterproof liners between layers. For example, one plastic produce bag between the inner and outer sock, and another between the outer sock and the boot, seals in sweat and keeps the insulating sock dry. Similarly, a plastic liner can go between glove liners and mitts. For the body, a thin waterproof shirt or jacket goes just over the synthetic underwear. Some people have more tolerance than others for the clammy feeling of vapor barrier liners, but they are seldom used during vigorous activity unless the temperature is well below freezing.

Putting It all together

When selecting cold weather clothing, bring along the other layers that you will be wearing with it, to make sure that they will fit together comfortably, and not bind or bunch when you move. If you will be snow camping, try lying down and turning over a few times, because you will probably be wearing at least some layers in the sleeping bag. Do the clothes stretch and move with you, or do they bind and shift? Cold weather clothing has not quite caught up with the natural insulation that caribou and wolves have evolved. But by knowing how clothing works, and selecting clothes that fit our activities as well as our bodies, we can survive and even enjoy winter weather.

Sleeping warm

Getting chilled at night can lower your resistance to hypothermia, altitude illness, and respiratory infections, as well as making you more susceptible to accidents the next day by reducing your physical and mental efficiency. So making sure that you sleep warmly and comfortably is good preventive medicine.

Preparing the ground

Before laying down your tent or ground cloth, remove any pebbles, twigs, or pine cones that could dig into you through your pad and bag. Remember the story of the princess and the pea. Avoid tall grass, because on a cool night it will collect a lot of dew, and so will your sleeping bag or shelter. Also avoid the bases of big gullies or descending valleys that can turn into wind tunnels as cold air flows down them at night.

If you can't find level ground, sleep with your head uphill. In a snow shelter, sleep on a shelf with a deeper trench beside it to collect and carry out the cold air. When digging a snow shelter in moderate temperatures, wear only your underwear under your waterproof outer layer. In colder temperatures, add only the minimum of synthetic layers to keep you warm while digging. Then put on more layers when you finish digging. If you tend to sleep on your back, a little padding under the sleeping pad at knee level will prevent hyper-extension of the knees.

Down sleeping bags

High quality goose down has the most loft of any sleeping bag fill, and so gives the most warmth for the weight. But it has two limitations: it collapses when wet; and because it is so compressible, it provides very little ground insulation under the body. As a result, you may need more thickness of foam pad underneath you than with a synthetic bag. Some down bags have shells of water-resistant but breathable fabric, which gives them considerable protection from both water and wind, but you still must be careful not to saturate them

from within. As a result, down bags work well in dry climates, but have little survival value in climates where they can get wet.

Synthetic sleeping bags

Synthetic bags are filled with fibers, usually polyester, that are crimped at a temperature of about $160°$ F to give them loft. They are heavier and bulkier than good down for the warmth they give. Also, they can lose loft if they are kept stuffed, especially in a hot car. The temperature inside a parked car or the trunk of a car driving on a hot summer day can be high enough to re-crimp synthetic fibers in the compressed position. And even if the fibers are not forcibly re-crimped, they lose their loft with use much faster than high-quality down. Transporting them in loose storage sacks, however, will extend their life. The advantage of synthetic bags is that the fibers do not absorb moisture, so they keep most of their loft and warmth even when the bag gets wet. Also, since they are less compressible than down, they provide more ground insulation.

Dressing for sleep

You can sleep warmer and get by with a lighter sleeping bag by wearing clothes inside it, but they need to be the right kind of clothes – stretchy synthetics. These clothes will not wrinkle or bind, and will also not absorb water from your sweat. An inner layer of synthetic underwear and a pullover or jacket of fleece or pile work well. Dry socks will keep your feet warm - it is impossible to feel warm if your feet are cold. A fleece cap or balaclava will prevent heat loss through your head. As you warm up inside the bag, you can remove layers of clothes.

In very cold weather, some people use vapor barrier liners (VBLs) inside their sleeping bags - bags of waterproof nylon that prevent evaporative heat loss by sweating and keep the moisture out of the insulation. The disadvantage is that VBLs may make you feel damp and clammy, even if you wear your synthetic underwear underneath.

Breath, fuel and water

When you breathe dry air, your circulatory system humidifies it with water from a network of blood vessels in the air passages, and you lose most that moisture when you exhale. If you breathe inside your bag, that water will soak into the bag's insulation. So you should keep your mouth and nose out of the bag, even when you cinch up the hood around your head.

Inside a tent, you should always have some back-to-front ventilation that will carry your warm, moist breath outside. Ideally, cold air comes in through the low vent at your feet and warmed moistened air rises to pass out the higher front vent. Otherwise moisture will condense on the tent fabric and rain down on your bag.

Digestion generates heat, so eating a good dinner will help keep you warm at night. You also need to be well hydrated, because dehydration can reduce blood volume. This in turn can slow down heat-generating metabolism and impair circulation to the hands and feet, making them feel cold. But if you let yourself get dehydrated all day then tank up before crawling into the sleeping bag, that guarantees some late night excursions to empty your bladder, which on a cold night can chill you down fast. Caffeine and alcohol before sleeping can also send you out with a full bladder, because they are diuretics.

Insulating pads

Closed cell foam pads are the most reliable ground insulation. Traditionally, they were just flat sections of foam, but now several models are available with patterns of ridges or nubbins that increase the effective insulation for the weight and bulk.

Thermarest® pads are inflatable, which adds insulating air to the foam inside. Their drawbacks are that they can be punctured and start leaking (so it is important to carry a patch) and the valve can fail. Also, the nylon shell is slippery, even if you spray it with an aerosol that makes it a bit tacky, so you can slide off it at night, especially if the ground under you is not quite level. The advantage is that it gives you much more insulation than a closed cell pad for its weight, and that it conforms more to your body, like a mattress. So it is less likely to impair circulation. For a very cold winter trip, a three-quarter length Thermarest® and a full-length closed cell foam pad is a good combination.

A small pillowcase of soft-textured nylon can be stuffed with any soft surplus clothing. Or you can make a pillow by zipping up a fleece or pile jacket, turning it inside out so that the sleeves are inside, then folding it with the zipper on the bottom.

Chapter 4. Wilderness wound care and bandaging

Photos courtesy of Ben Schifrin, MD

In both wilderness and urban situations, you need to stop serious bleeding immediately and protect yourself from possible blood-borne diseases. In the wilderness, even minor wounds can easily become infected and turn into major emergencies if you do not treat them properly. So wilderness rescuers also need to know how to clean wounds and keep them clean with effective dressings and bandages.

Stopping the leak

The best way to stop serious bleeding is to squeeze the leaking blood vessels by pressing firmly on the wound, using thick dressings, a clean bandana, or a gloved hand to apply direct pressure; then replace manual pressure with a pressure bandage. If that doesn't stop the bleeding completely, then for an injury in a limb you can supplement the direct pressure with a tourniquet. Dressings with hemostatic agents can help control bleeding, but they are expensive.

When is bleeding serious?

Blood from a cut artery spurts with every contraction of the left ventricle, until blood volume and blood pressure drop. So until arterial bleeding is controlled, it can prevent the formation of a clot. Bleeding from a cut vein does not spurt, and is therefore usually easier to control; but if it is more than a trickle, the patient can still lose enough blood to go into shock. Clotting, the body's mechanism for sealing an open wound, can take 10 minutes or more even for minor wounds.

Tourniquets

To apply a commercial tourniquet, put it around the limb an inch or two proximal to the wound (but never on a joint), and pull the webbing through the buckle until it is tight. Then twist the attached rod to increase the pressure until the bleeding stops and there is no distal pulse, and secure the rod. Arterial bleeding will stop when the compression equals systolic blood pressure, and there is no distal pulse. Even for severe venous bleeding, however, you should tighten the tourniquet until there is no distal pulse. Otherwise,

arterial blood can continue to flow into the limb and be trapped, causing compartment syndrome.

You can improvise a tourniquet with a folded triangular bandage or other strong piece of cloth. After tying it snugly around the limb, pass a stick through the knot, twist the stick until bleeding stops, and secure the stick with the tails of the bandage. After applying a tourniquet, you should write a large T on the patient's forehead with a sharpie pen, as well as the time applied. Once applied, a tourniquet should not be loosened or removed.

Protecting yourself

Blood may carry disease organisms such as hepatitis B or C, so you should protect your hands with gloves and your eyes with goggles, if necessary.

For many years, latex, made from the sap of a tropical tree, was the standard for impermeable gloves that are also light and flexible. Unfortunately latex contains proteins that can cause allergic reactions. Even a minor allergic reaction can cause the skin to crack, scale, or blister. Although rare, a severe reaction can cause anaphylactic shock, which is often fatal. Because of the growing allergy problem, latex is being phased out of the health care industry. Synthetic gloves, however, give the same protection without risk of allergy. The standard synthetic alternative to latex is nitrile.

Preventing infection

A healthy immune system can usually protect living tissue in minor wounds if they are not too dirty. But it does not protect dead tissue or foreign matter. These become colonization sites for bacteria, which can then multiply until they overwhelm the body's defenses. So the only way to prevent infection in the wilderness is to clean the wound and keep it clean. And the only safe way to clean an open wound in the field is to irrigate it with a forceful jet of water. This may not be pleasant for the patient, but it is essential for preventing infection.

Wound irrigation syringes with blunt needles are sold by several wilderness medical supply companies

They produce 7-10 psi (pounds per square inch) of pressure. To avoid splashback, you can run the syringe or the needle through the bottom of a plastic cup or something else that will act as a shield.

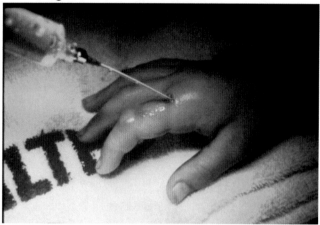

A plastic squeeze bottle with a screw-on cap that has a narrow opening for squirting out a thin stream of liquid can also be used for wound irrigation. Another alternative is a large heavy-duty ziplock bag with a pinhole in the bottom corner. Just fill it up, seal the top, and squeeze. However, it will not produce nearly as much pressure as a syringe. Whatever device you use, keep irrigating until the wound is as clean as you can get it. Disinfected water from your water bottle is ideal, but use the cleanest water available.

If you see dirt or debris embedded in the wound that does not flush out, then you need to pick it out with clean tweezers. After removing the debris, irrigate again. Lacerations from a clean knife or other sharp object are least likely to become infected, because they leave relatively little crushed dead tissue in the wound.

Puncture wounds are at high risk of infection, because they may carry contaminants deep into the tissues and are hard to clean. If possible, apply hot compresses to a puncture wound (20 minutes every 2 hours) for a day or two, to draw out contaminants.

Disinfectants and "antibiotic" ointments

Antiseptics will not completely disinfect a wound, but they may slow down bacterial growth. Povidone-iodine (a buffered 10% iodine solution) and benzalkonium chloride are the two standard antiseptics (Greek *anti* "against" + *sepsis* "putrefaction") for hospital and emergency care use. They also come in sealed antiseptic towelettes, which are good for scrubbing the skin around a wound and for cleaning your hands if water is short. To carry either solution in your kit, use a

2 oz. plastic squeeze bottle with a hinged squirt nozzle in the cap. Wrap the threads with Teflon tape (found in the plumbing section of hardware stores) to prevent leaking. Tincture of iodine, mercurochrome, and hydrogen peroxide are no longer recommended, because they may cause some tissue damage; and alcohol doesn't work.

Honey has been used in wound dressings for thousands of years. Many studies have shown that it is effective, even on organisms that are resistant to antibiotics. Dark manucca honey from New Zealand (Medihoney) has been approved for medical use because it has an especially high level of anti-microbial activity. But all unprocessed honey reduces wound infection and promotes healing by several mechanisms. The sugar dehydrates bacteria by drawing out the fluid osmotically across cell membranes. Since honey is acidic, it disrupts the membranes of gram negative bacteria. And an enzyme in dark, unprocessed honey (glucose oxidase) releases a low level of hydrogen peroxide (not enough to cause tissue damage). Honey also helps keeps the wound moist, which promotes healing.

Much of what is sold as honey in stores, however, is imported and mixed with high fructose corn syrup. Moreover, some imported honey is contaminated with lead and animal antibiotics. So it is best to buy locally produced unprocessed honey for both nutritional and medicinal purposes.

Antibiotic ointments are widely used in hospitals and first aid kits, but they do not actually kill bacteria. They may help to protect against infection by forming a barrier, but so will any ointment. Another problem with antibiotic ointments is that they may cause allergic reactions. So there is no substitute for irrigating a wound thoroughly, and then keeping it clean, especially in the wilderness.

Signs of infection

If bacteria in a wound are increasing and multiplying, the body responds in several ways. It sends chemicals to the area that increase circulation (so that the skin around the wound becomes red) and that loosen the bonds between cells in blood vessel walls. White blood cells slip out of the blood vessels to attack and devour the bacteria. Fluid accumulates, causing swelling, which causes pain by putting pressure on nerves. The swollen wound site will also be pressure-sensitive. All the chemical activity produces heat, so the area around the wound will feel warm. Fluid with dead white blood cells (pus) may leak out of the wound.

If the infection spreads, you may see red streaks going towards the heart, as dead red blood cells and other debris drain through the lymph vessels. Lymph vessels have filters or nodes that remove solids from the fluid, so these nodes may swell. Large lymph nodes are in the armpits and groin, for example. Another reaction of the body to spreading infection is fever - raising the temperature may make the body slightly less hospitable to some bacteria and viruses.

If a wound is showing signs of infection, the body probably needs help to overcome it. Hot soaks will draw pus out of the wound, but the patient may need an oral antibiotic. Since this is a prescription drug, you would need to evacuate the patient to a hospital unless you had a doctor with a supply of antibiotics on the trip. Alternatively, you could have every trip member bring his or her own prescribed oral antibiotic just in case of emergencies.

Closing the wound

Any wound large enough to require evacuation, or showing signs of infection, should be left open in the field unless it must be closed to control bleeding.

If you decide to close a clean minor wound, the simplest way is with butterfly bandages. You can make your own butterflies out of athletic or adhesive tape, or duct tape for a large wound. Just make a center section non-sticky by cutting part way in from the edges and folding them over. Before applying tape, dry the skin around the wound with sterile gauze. Stick one or more pieces of tape to one side of the wound, use the other ends to pull the wound shut, and stick them down.

Wound healing

As the first step in wound healing, the blood delivers thrombin and fibrinogen, proteins that forms a matrix of fibers in the wound. This matrix forms a clot that stops bleeding, and provides a framework into which living cells can migrate, from the bottom of the wound up, pushing the fibrous material toward the surface to form a scab.

Some types of wounds heal more easily than others. A clean, straight cut made with a sharp edge is easy to align, and will usually close without complications if you keep it clean. A jagged cut with crushed tissue is less likely to heal by itself. Also, wound healing slows down at high altitude, because even when you are acclimatized, the blood delivers less oxygen to the tissues than at sea level. Above about 18,000 feet, without supplemental oxygen, wound healing stops.

Another problem with wounds outdoors is that the very parts of your body most likely to be injured, because you use them so much, are for the same reason hard to keep clean - especially the hands and feet.

Types of wounds

Different mechanisms of injury can cause different kinds of damage. A sliding fall or skid can scrape off layers of skin. Granite rash from sliding down a rock slope, or road rash from a bicycling accident, are typical. Abrasions (from Latin *abradere*, "to scrape off, to shave") tend to be painful because of the number of nerve endings affected, and laborious to clean if grit or dirt is ground into the damaged skin. Also, a small first aid kit is unlikely to have enough sterile dressings to cover and protect a large abrasion.

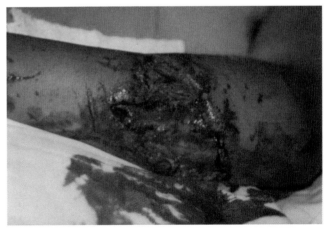

Wound caused by abrasion, deep enough to damage underlying tissues.

Lacerations (from Latin *laceratio*, "a tearing or mangling") can damage underlying structures as well as skin, such as large blood vessels, nerves, tendons, muscles, or bones. Once you have treated the wound, you should check distal functions for the effects of any damage: circulation, sensation, and movement (CSM).

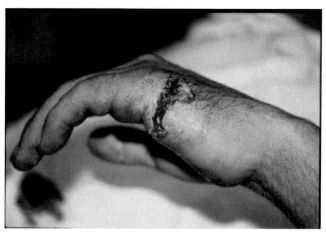
Laceration

Avulsions (from Latin *avulsus*, past participle of *avulsere*, "to pull away, tear off") are wounds in which living tissue is partially or completely torn away. If there is no serious bleeding, avulsed tissue that is not completely separated can be bandaged in its normal position after cleaning.

Amputations (from Latin *amputatio*, "a pruning") are probably the most dramatic of wounds, and you might have to use a tourniquet to control bleeding. After controlling the bleeding, wrap the amputated part in sterile gauze, and seal it in a water-tight plastic bag. Keep the bag cool during evacuation by putting it in ice, if available. Otherwise, wrap the bag in thick cloths and keep the cloths wet.

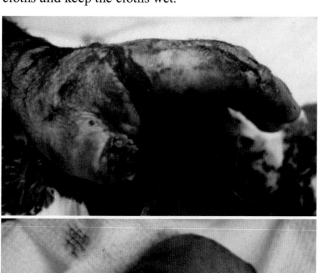

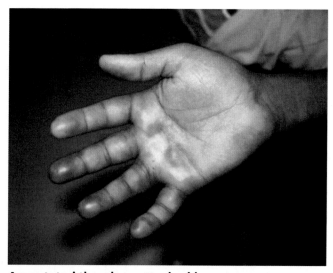
Amputated thumb, reattached by a surgeon

Bandages and dressings

Bandages ("to bind") hold dressings in place. Dressings "dress" a wound, protecting it from further contamination. A scab is no barrier to bacteria, so the wound still needs to be protected. If possible, dressings should be sterile.

For serious bleeding, you need bulky dressings to soak up blood and help form a clot. For other wounds, especially burns, non-stick dressings are best. You can secure a small dressing with tape. There are many specialized dressings with attached adhesive strips or bandage tails, ranging from the small band aid to the thick battle dressing developed by the military, which can quickly be tied to any part of the body. To remove tape and stuck dressings painlessly, lift up a corner and start dabbing the adhesive with an alcohol wipe. If hair is under the tape, pull in the direction that the hair is oriented (e.g., toward the hand or foot on a limb). The alcohol will dissolve the adhesive as you peel the tape. Non-stretchy bandages are good for applying quick pressure to stop bleeding. Stretchy gauze roller bandages conform to the body, so they are good for holding dressings on wounds that just need to be protected from contamination. For finger bandages, the 2" width is convenient, and the 4" width works for bandaging other parts of the body. Surgical roller bandages are also stretchy and cling to themselves. Elastic bandages are stronger, used mostly to wrap swollen joints. Injuries can kill people in two ways: by damaging or destroying vital organs outright; or by interfering with the delivery of oxygen and other substances to the vital organs by the circulating blood.

Shock

If the vital organs are not getting enough oxygen to maintain themselves, they start to die. This condition is called shock. It can happen in several ways. But even though the initial signs and symptoms may differ, the final effect is the same. A rescuer's first priority, after taking care of the ABCs and scene safety, is usually to prevent or minimize shock.

Mechanisms of shock

How can injuries interfere with oxygen delivery?

- Loss of blood volume can cause **hypovolemic shock** ("too little volume"). Blood volume can be depleted by severe external or internal bleeding (**hemorrhagic shock**), or by severe dehydration.
- Circulation will become sluggish if a cervical spine injury or a neurotoxin cuts off signals from the brain that increase heart rate and constrict blood vessels (**neurogenic shock**). The arteries will dilate, causing blood to pool.
- Damage to the heart from a heart attack that blocks blood supply to part of the heart muscle (**cardiogenic shock**) will also reduce circulation by making the pump less efficient.
- Allergic reaction to intrusion of a foreign protein (**anaphylactic shock**) will reduce the supply of air to the lungs by constricting airways and make circulation sluggish by dilating the arteries.
- An infection that spreads through the whole body can do so much damage to blood vessels that they leak fluid into surrounding tissues (**septic shock**).

Treating for shock

In many cases, you can prevent or at least minimize shock by identifying and treating the cause:

- Stop serious bleeding from an open wound.
- Reduce pain and prevent further damage by splinting a fracture.
- Prevent further damage if you find signs and symptoms of a spinal injury. See the section on spinal injury management in the chapter on specific injuries.
- Help a heart attack victim to take prescribed medications and avoid exertion while waiting for evacuation. See the section on heart attack in the chapter on medical problems in the wilderness.

- Help someone with an allergic reaction take prescribed medications.
- Prevent infection. If infection spreads enough to cause septic shock, the patient has little chance of survival.

Do not wait for signs and symptoms of shock to appear. In a wilderness situation, there are four important things that you can do:

- Guard the patient's airway, since shock victims may be nauseated and level of responsiveness may be going down. Vomiting and aspirating the vomit into the lungs is always a danger. Position the patient so that vomit will not go into the lungs – leaning forward if sitting, or in the recovery (left lateral) position if lying down.
- Give oxygen if you have it, since the main with shock is shortage of oxygen in the vital organs.
- Maintain body temperature with ground insulation and covers, since any problem with oxygen delivery slows down metabolism and heat production.
- Give psychological support and reassurance, since the patient's emotional state affects functions controlled by the autonomic nervous system, which can make shock more or less severe.

Hypovolemic shock

If bleeding or severe dehydration reduces the blood volume, the circulatory system will usually compensate in several ways. So long as compensation works, the circulatory system may continue to deliver enough blood and oxygen to the vital organs to keep them alive. If the circulation cannot fully compensate, however, or compensation begins to fail, vital organs will also begin to fail. Then you will see much more ominous signs and symptoms. So it is important to recognize when vital systems are stressed and to support them promptly.

Compensation for hypovolemic shock varies depending on age and physical fitness. A healthy child may compensate so well that you will not realize the problem until compensation fails. Then the child's condition can get worse very fast. Elderly people however, especially those with poor circulation or limited lung capacity, have much less margin to compensate for loss of blood volume. Therefore, you may see the effects of poor circulation and oxygen shortage in the elderly much more quickly.

An adult has about a quart of blood (a little less than a liter) for every 25 pounds of body weight, so a 150-pound adult has about six quarts of blood, of which about half is liquid. How do you tell if somebody has lost a significant amount of blood?

You can get a good idea of lost blood volume from the effects on the patient.

- Circulation withdraws from skin to concentrate on vital organs, so skin gets cool and pale. In dark-skinned persons, check the gums. Skin may also get sweaty, because that is part of the body's automatic fight or flight reaction.
- Respiration speeds up to blow off accumulating carbon dioxide in the blood and becomes shallow when the chest does not have time to expand or contract fully.
- The patient may feel anxious and agitated because of the adrenaline coursing through the system.

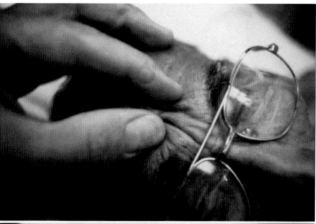

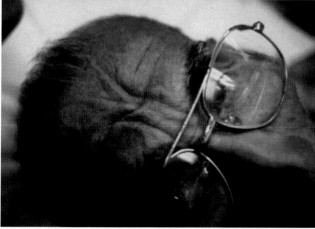

In severe dehydration, the skin loses elasticity, so that it remains tented when pinched.

As shock progresses and the body continues compensating:

- Pulse becomes weak because of reduced blood volume and rapid because the heart speeds up to compensate.
- Blood pressure may drop, because blood volume is down and circulation is withdrawn from the limbs.
- Pulse may speed up significantly, and blood pressure drop further, after the patient sits or stands up, especially in the elderly (postural hypotension).
- Capillary refill (when you press on the nail bed or forehead) may slow down - it takes longer for the pink to come back.
- Pupils dilate (the relaxed position of the iris muscles) because of reduced blood flow and respond more slowly to light.
- Nausea and thirst signal the withdrawal of circulation from the digestive system.
- Urine production decreases or stops.
- Weakness and possibly trembling in the arms and legs signals withdrawal of circulation from the muscles.
- Level of responsiveness drops because of poor circulation to the brain, and the patient usually becomes disoriented.

If compensation and your efforts to support the vital systems fail:

- Skin will become mottled (from patchy, pooled blood) and cold, and sweating may stop.
- Pulse will be fast, and you may not feel it.
- Blood pressure may not register.
- Breathing will be agonal (gasping and irregular).
- The patient will soon become unresponsive.

A patient who has lost 25% or less of the total blood volume will usually be given crystalloid by paramedics to replace the liquid part of the blood. This patient will continue to need oxygen, because it will take time for the body to replace lost red blood cells. A patient who has lost 30% or more of the blood volume will have a very weak pulse and need a transfusion.

Bandaging with gauze rollers

To bandage an arm or leg, start on the narrow end of the limb, distal to the wound, and wrap up-limb. The following drawing shows a figure 8 spiral, which puts more uniform pressure on a bleeding wound. Angle the roller alternately up-limb and down-limb about 20° with every other wrap. The interlocking pattern makes a secure bandage that will stay in place as the patient uses the limb.

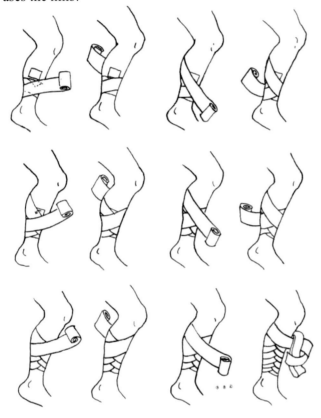

- Leave one corner of the gauze sticking out on the first wrap, then fold it over and lock it down with the second wrap. This anchors the bandage.
- Hold the roller so that it unrolls onto the limb and maintain even tension as you wrap.
- When you have almost covered the dressing, fold the last exposed corner of it over the gauze roller and lock the dressing down with the next wrap.
- Continue wrapping well past the dressing.
- To tie off, fold the roller back over your finger so that you have a single end and a double end to tie together. If you don't have enough roller left, tape it to itself.

If you are improvising a roller bandage from a strip of non-stretchy cloth, use a reverse spiral to cinch the down-limb edge of the bandage. For a reverse spiral, do a half-turn toward the narrower end of the limb with every wrap.

To bandage a wound on the point of the elbow or knee, anchor the gauze roller distal to the joint. Then, holding the dressing in place with your other hand, angle the bandage diagonally across the dressing and wrap the bandage around the limb proximal to the joint. Diagonal back across the dressing, locking down its corner and making an X, then do another wrap around the limb distal to the joint

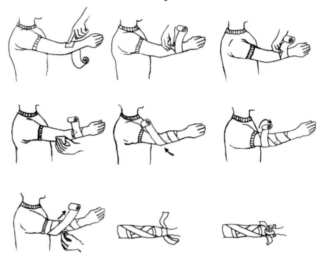

To bandage a wound on the hand with a gauze roller, anchor it at the wrist, and wrap diagonally to the hand to secure the dressing.

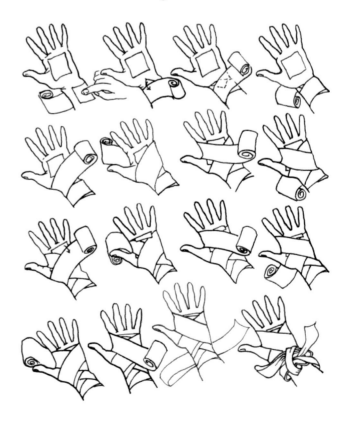

If the wound is in the hollow of the palm, add some extra layers of dressing or clean cloth to fill the hollow so that the bandage will exert pressure on the dressing. After covering and securing the dressing, wrap diagonally back to the wrist in the other direction to make an X. and tie off the bandage at the wrist.

For a severely bleeding hand wound, fill the hand with several rollers or other padding (after applying sterile dressing) so that the patient's fingers wrap around the padding in the relaxed position of function, with the tip of the thumb even with the tip of the index finger, then anchor a gauze roller at the wrist, and wrap it diagonally around the loose fist to hold the fingers in place. This is also a good soft splint for a smashed hand or multiple fractured fingers.

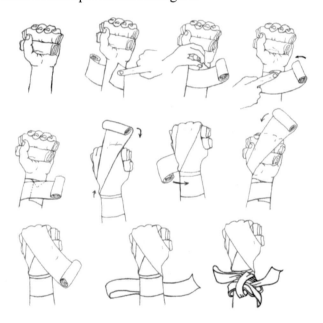

To do a good finger bandage:
- Wrap a dressing around the injured finger, separating the fingers with dressings if several are injured.
- Anchor a gauze roller at the wrist, wrapping in the direction that will take the roller diagonally across the back of the hand to the injured finger, so that closing the hand will tighten rather than loosen the bandage. If the little finger or ring finger is injured, for example, the wrap starts from the thumb side of the wrist.
- Spiral up and back down the finger(s) to secure the dressing. If the fingertip is injured, secure the dressing over the tip with some up and down wraps, then anchor them with more spiral wraps.

- From the base of the finger, inside, bring the roller back to the wrist and anchor it.

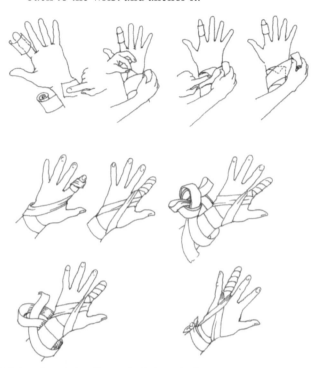

If the tip of the finger is injured, do some up and down wraps to hold part of the dressing over the tip and secure them with more spiral wraps before anchoring the bandage at the wrist.

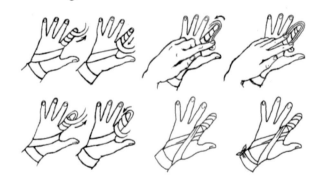

To bandage any part of the head or face, a gauze roller also works, but you may have to alternate vertical and horizontal wraps to make it secure. When going around the back of the head, be sure to pass below the bump at the base of the skull so that the bandage won't slip off.

A figure 8 roller bandage can also secure a dressing to a wound on any part of the foot, including the sole. Anchor the bandage at the ankle, then wrap it over the top of the foot and around the sole, capturing the dressing. Wrap diagonally back over the top of the foot and around the ankle. With the next wrap around the sole of the foot, lock a corner of the dressing, and continue to wrap until the wound is securely covered.

If there is not enough bandage left to tie it off, tape the end of the bandage to itself.

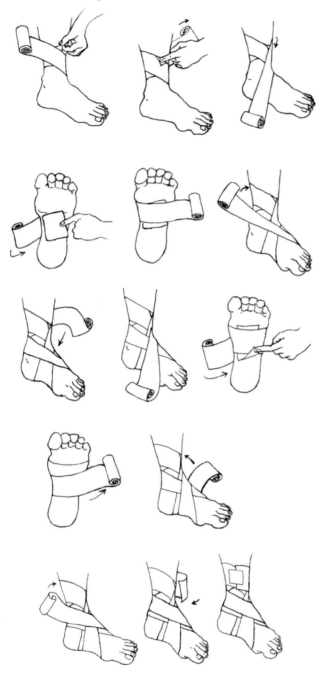

Making a triangular bandage

Use cotton muslin or any other fabric that is not slippery or bulky. Scavenge old bed sheets, or go to a fabric store. Start with a square 40" on a side (or 42" for a large bandage). Cut on the diagonal. For durable bandages, hem the edges.

Folding the triangle into a cravat

For most bandages, you need to fold the cravat. If you have a clean surface on which to lay it out, fold the point to the long side and continue folding it in half until it is the width that you want. If you are outdoors, you can use a technique that requires a little practice

- Drape the long side over the fingers of your left hand and the point over the fingers of your right hand, keeping your thumbs out.
- Flip the center outward, clapping your hands.
- With your left thumb, clamp the cloth hanging inside your right fingers.
- Reach out to the end of the fold with your right hand and pinch grip the cloth.
- Now flip the cloth outward with your left thumb as you pull your right hand toward you.

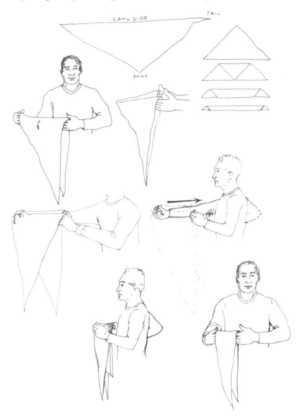

Bandaging with cravats

To bandage with a cravat, maintain the tension as you wrap. To control bleeding with a pressure bandage, capture the dressing with the center of the bandage, wrap the tails around the limb a few times, then tie them together right over the dressing so that the knot puts extra pressure on the wound. Always use a square knot. You can use the same pressure bandage to hold a dressing on the forehead, making sure that the tails pass below the bump at the base of the skull so that the bandage doesn't slip off.

Square knot & quick release

To tie a square knot, the mnemonic is: Right over left, left over right. In the following picture, the right tail has gone over the left (and around and through). Then the tail on the left goes over the tail on the right (and around and through). If you look at the resulting knot (top right), you'll see that it is square and symmetrical – two U-shaped bends of the cravat intersecting each other. To do a quick release, pull one tail away from the standing end until it straightens out, converting the square knot into a slip knot. Then slip the knot off.

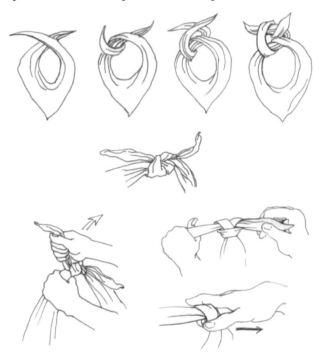

For a scalp wound, you can hold dressings in place with a turban bandage.

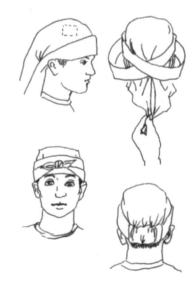

Lay the triangle over the head with the point hanging down behind. Position the long side just above the eyebrows, and wrap the two tails around the head, crossing just below the bump at the base of the skull. Then bring the tails around and tie them in front. Now grip the point of the cravat that is hanging down the back and tug it till the bandage is snug over the scalp. Finally, tuck in the excess.

Hypovolemic shock

If bleeding or severe dehydration reduces the blood volume, the circulatory system will usually compensate in several ways. Circulation withdraws from the skin to concentrate on vital organs, so the skin gets cool and pale. In dark-skinned persons, check the gums. Skin may also get sweaty, part of the body's automatic fight or flight reaction triggered by the release of adrenaline, which may also make the patient feel anxious and agitated. Respiration speeds up to blow off accumulating carbon dioxide in the blood and becomes shallow when the chest does not have time to expand or contract fully.

As shock progresses, pulse may become weak from loss of blood volume, and more rapid to compensate. Nausea and thirst signal the withdrawal of circulation from the digestive system. Weakness and possible trembling in the arms and legs signal withdrawal of circulation from the muscles. Pupils may dilate and respond more slowly to light, and level of responsiveness drops because of poor circulation to the brain. If compensation fails, skin becomes mottled and cold from patchy pooled blood, pulse may be impalpable, and breathing irregular. The patient will soon become unresponsive.

To treat or prevent hypovolemic shock, first control bleeding. Have the patient lie down and maintain body temperature, since reduced circulation and delivery of oxygen and nutrients will reduce metabolism and heat production. Give oxygen if available, and protect the airway if the patient becomes nauseated. Psychological support and reassurance (as described in the first chapter) can help stabilize functions controlled by the autonomic nervous system. But elevating the legs is no longer recommended because there is no evidence that it improves circulation to vital organs, and it could aggravate fractures or internal injuries.

Compensation for hypovolemic shock varies with age and fitness. A child may seem stable until compensation fails. Then the child's condition can get worse very fast. Elderly people however, especially those with poor circulation or limited lung capacity, have much less margin to compensate for loss of blood volume. Therefore, you usually see the effects of poor circulation and oxygen shortage in the elderly much more quickly.

Preventing foot blisters

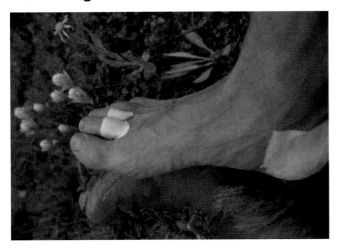

As your feet move around inside your boots, friction on the outer layer of skin can shear it from the underlying layer, and as fluid accumulates between the separated layers, you grow blisters. Prevent blisters by:
- Proper boot fitting.
- Padding boots to fill gaps and cover rough edges.
- The 2-sock system (plus a cushioned insole).
- Covering hot spots (or potential hot spots) with Moleskin or tape before they grow into blisters.

When fitting boots, wear thin synthetic inner socks that cling like an extra layer of skin, and thick socks of wool or synthetic. With the boots unlaced, you should be able to slide your foot forward enough to fit two or three fingers in the space behind your heel. After lacing up the boots, test them:
- Walk around in them. Do deep leg stretches. Jump. Jog in place. Any pressure? Excessive heel lift?
- Stand on the inclined surface of a fitting stool, toes down. Do your toes slide forward and touch the fronts of the boots? If so, the boots are too loose.
- Plant one foot on the incline with the toes up and step up. Does your heel lift more than a fraction of an inch? If so, you have too much heel slop.

If your boots already have heel slop or rough edges inside, pad them with Mole Foam (adhesive cloth with foam padding). Make sure your boots are clean and dry, cut Mole Foam to fit, and press the adhesive firmly onto the leather. Going uphill, heel lift may cause blisters, so cover your heels and Achilles tendons with large pieces of Moleskin or tape to protect them from friction. Before going downhill, tighten your laces so that your toes don't slide forward, and tape toes likely to get blisters.

Treating blisters

Once blisters have formed, you can try to prevent them from popping or puncture them. If a blister on the heel or side of the foot is still small:
- Cut a donut of mole foam to fit around the blister and take the pressure off it.
- Lay a piece of Spenco 2nd Skin® on the blister, fitting inside the hole.

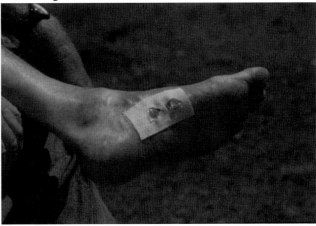

- Cover the donut with Moleskin or tape, sealing in the 2nd Skin.

If a blister has started to form on the bottom of the foot, any thick covering would make walking uncomfortable. So the best way to protect the incipient blister from friction is with a large piece of duct tape - put a small piece of duct tape in the center of the sticky side, so that the tape will not stick to the blister.

To puncture a blister, sterilize a needle in a flame and pierce the blister at the base. You may need to enlarge the hole to prevent it from re-sealing and the blister from filling up again. Let the blister drain, irrigate, and disinfect it as you would any open wound. Afterwards, use the same technique described above to protect it against further abrasion.

Burns

Photos courtesy of Ben Schifrin, MD.

In the wilderness, the most common cause of burns is cooking accidents. This includes minor burns to the hands from grabbing hot metal; potentially major burns from stove flare-ups; and scalds from tipping over pots of boiling liquid. If you cook in a tent, flare-ups can start a fire, even though tent fabrics are supposed to be flame retardant. Wildfires are the other way to get burned in the wilderness.

Avoiding and preventing wildfires

If you build campfires in the wilderness, do it on mineral soil, not soil that is blended with decaying forest vegetation and threaded with roots from surrounding trees. Fire can work its way down through vegetation debris to tree roots and travel along the roots. Careless campers have awakened to find that the surrounding trees had turned into giant torches.

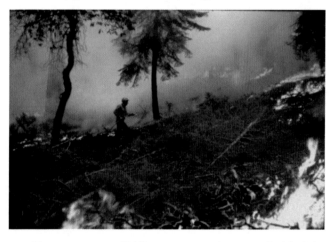

To escape a wildfire, you need to get behind it. You can't outrun a wind-driven fire, especially if it is going uphill. Wind flowing upslope compresses the layer of moving air, which increases its velocity. Also, smoke and superheated gases are pushed up ahead of the fire, especially through gullies (natural ascent routes), which act like the flume of a fireplace. In hilly terrain with narrow valleys between ridges, fire can even jump from crest to crest.

But fire needs fuel. In a shallow fuel area, such as grassland, fire will burn through fast, and you may be able to get behind it through a gap. But forest fires, especially in areas that have accumulated a lot of deadwood because of fire control, burn long and deep.

If you can't get around or through them, or find a large bare area, your only hope may be to jump in a stream or lake. Heat moves upward, so the water will keep you cool, though you need to get as far as possible from a fire to breathe relatively clean, oxygenated air.

Thermal burn factors and damage

Thermal burns can be caused by exposure to flames, contact with a hot object, scalding by hot liquid, or steam. Burn damage depends on the temperature and conductivity of the heat source, contact time, and contact area. Hot liquid or metal can cause a much more serious burn than an open flame of the same temperature, because they transmit heat much faster than air. However, chefs can plunge their hands into boiling water for a second without harm. But an elderly person trapped in a bathtub can suffer serious burns in water at a temperature as low as 113° F, because of greater contact time and contact area. Firewalkers can walk barefoot over a bed of porous red-hot charcoal if they don't stumble, but they would not last long if they tried the same stunt on a red-hot griddle of iron, which conducts heat much more efficiently.

Burns can damage or destroy one or more layers of skin directly by heat. The inflammatory response of the body then causes accumulation of fluid to the burn, which raises blisters in a partial thickness burn. When a large part of the skin is damaged or destroyed, fluid can ooze out and dehydrate the patient. The human body is about two-thirds water, and one function of skin is to hold it in.

Serious burns over 10% of an adult's body would evaporate about a liter per day; and serious burns over half the body area would leak and evaporate 4-5 liters of water per day. Each liter of water that evaporates from a burn takes away about 570 Kilocalories of heat, which is as much heat as the body produces in an hour of vigorous activity. So a burn patient can easily become hypothermic as well as dehydrated.

The smoke and heated gases from fires can damage the air passages and lungs if inhaled, and cause the most deaths in burn victims. Inhalation injuries are most common in enclosed spaces, but can happen in forest fires or accidents inside a tent. Carbon monoxide (produced by all fires) can be deadly even in low concentrations, and burning synthetic fabric gives off hydrogen cyanide. Steam can burn not only the air passages but also the lungs, because water vapor has more heat capacity than air and is more conductive.

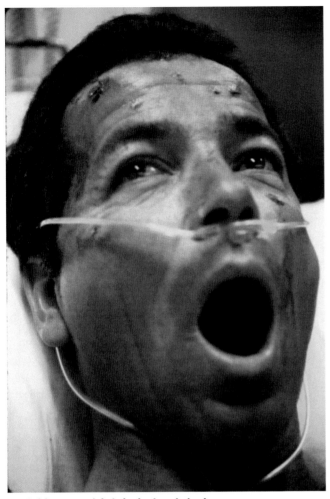

Facial burns with inhalation injuries

Serious burns also put stress on vital organs. Shortage of blood and oxygen can cause ulcers in the stomach. Kidneys can be overloaded with proteins dumped in the blood from damaged tissues. And fluid can leak into the lungs because of damage from inhalation injuries. Also, since the skin is a barrier against microorganisms, serious burns leave the patient open to infection, which may develop within days.

Assessing thermal burns

Most textbooks give the rule of nines for estimating the percentage of skin area covered by burns. Each major part of the body (e.g., an arm or the front of the torso) has either 9% or 18% of the total skin area. There are two problems with this rule: it is hard to remember, and burns seldom neatly cover one part of the body completely. So the rule of ones is much more useful. The patient's hand, from wrist fold to fingertips but

excluding the thumb, is about 1% of the patient's total skin area. So estimate how many hands of skin the burn covers.

If a burn is superficial, skin will redden because of increased circulation to the injury, but it will turn white when you press on it (forcing the blood away), then turn red again as the circulation comes back. Superficial burns may not require dressings because the living layers of skin are intact. Only the transparent, non-living outer layer may peel off.

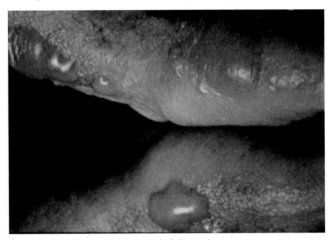

Partial thickness burn with blistering

In a partial thickness burn, several layers of skin are seriously damaged, and the rush of circulation to the damaged layers pushes them apart to form blisters. These burns are extremely painful, because the damage triggers so many nerve endings.

Full thickness burns do not hurt because all tissues in the skin, including nerves, have been killed. The skin may be charred, deep red, or white; or it may be burned away, exposing deeper tissues. Full thickness burns may be surrounded by partial thickness burns, however, which will hurt.

How do you decide whether a burn requires evacuation? Any full thickness burn is serious; and any partial thickness burn that covers more than 5% of the total skin area, or any significant part of the face, hands or genitals, requires evacuation. Even a superficial burn may be serious enough to require evacuation if it covers more than 20% of the skin area. When in doubt, the patient's condition should make your decision clear. A burned patient who is shivering, vomiting, or feverish urgently needs to be evacuated.

Burns that impair function are also more serious. Facial burns can affect the eyes, and inhalation of smoke or superheated gasses can affect the airway and

47

lungs. A circumferential burn to a limb can impair distal circulation. And any serious burn to the hand or foot can cause permanent loss of function.

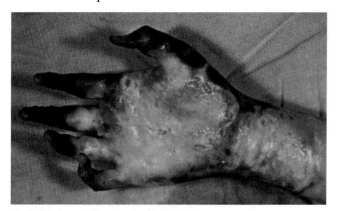

Full thickness burns to fingers

Treating thermal burns

Immediate care for a thermal burn is to stop the burning by removing the patient from the source of heat; then cool the burned area with water. If clothes are burning, smother the flame. If scalding liquid is saturating clothing, get the clothing off immediately, because it will still be broiling the victim's skin. Then cool the skin with water, because (like a roast just out of the oven) it will still be cooking.

In the wilderness, your first concern after cooling the burn will be pain control. An expedition doctor would probably give morphine to someone with a severe burn. Over the counter painkillers are not as effective, but you should use the strongest that you have if a burn patient is in severe pain.

A non-stick dressing is best for a burn. If you do not have any, you can use a moist dressing on any burn less than about 10% of total body area. It will be more soothing than a dry dressing. For a larger burn, however, a wet dressing could chill the patient into hypothermia. Change the dressing regularly

After pain control, your next problem with a serious, extensive burn is fluid loss. If the patient is alert enough and not too nauseated to swallow safely, you should provide fluids with electrolytes (runner's drink or Oral Rehydration Salts, diluted to half-strength) and make sure that the patient drinks regularly. An occlusive dressing, made by taping a piece of plastic over a regular dressing, may reduce fluid loss as well as preventing further contamination of the injury through the dressing.

Electrical burns

Electricity, like other forms of energy, follows the path of least resistance. Nerves, blood, and muscle are more than half water, so they are good conductors of electricity. Bone, fat, and dry skin (especially calloused skin) have less water, so they are more resistant. If your body becomes part of an electrical circuit, the current flowing through it can cause serious damage by heating the tissues. Damage depends on the voltage and current, as well as the duration of contact and which part of the body it goes through.

Voltage is the potential difference in electrical energy between two points in a circuit. According to **Ohm's Law**: Voltage = Current times Resistance. So the greater the resistance, the more voltage it will take to force a given current through. Current is measured in amperes (amps).

Household circuits in the United States are usually 110 volts and 15 to 20 amps, though some appliances require 220 volts. This voltage usually causes only contact burns. Industrial voltage (over 500 volts) can cause severe damage to muscles and organs as the current flows through the body, which will not be apparent from the entrance and exit wounds. It can also cause **cardiac arrest** if the current crosses the chest or **respiratory arrest** if the current affects the respiratory center of the brain. Power cords in household and industrial circuits are insulated with material that has high resistance, so they can be safely handled. High tension power lines, however (20,000-100,000 volts) are insulated only by air. Current from power lines can arc through the air, creating its own conductive pathway of ions, to make you part of the circuit. So it is not safe even to approach a downed power line.

Direct current (DC), which was championed by Thomas Edison, flows in one direction. Contact with it usually causes a single muscle contraction that can blow the patient away from the source. But most power is transmitted by alternating current (AC), which changes direction 60 times per second, because AC (based on inventions by Nicola Tesla) can be stepped up to very high voltages and transmitted over long distances with little power loss. Contact with AC can cause sustained muscle contraction that can lock the patient on to the electrical source.

Never touch a patient who may still be in contact with an electrical source until the current is turned off.

Remember that electrical burns, especially from industrial current, will have both entrance and exit wounds, which should both be covered with dry sterile dressings. Give oxygen if you have it, and check for any breathing problems or irregular pulse.

Chemical burns

Some chemicals can damage skin and underlying tissues on contact. Strong acids break down proteins in cells and solidify the tissues into a scab, which can limit penetration. Since the damage resembles the damage of thermal burns, injuries from contact with strong chemicals are also called burns. Strong bases liquefy skin and underlying tissues, so they can penetrate more easily into underlying tissues. Strength of acids and bases is measured by the pH (power of hydrogen) scale, since their reactions involve the exchange of hydrogen ions (protons). Acids give up protons, and bases bind protons. The strongest acids have a pH of 1; the strongest bases a pH of 14. Pure water has a pH of 7, which is neutral. Skin has a pH between 5 and 6, which is just slightly acidic.

Sulphuric acid is found in some toilet bowl and drain cleaners, as well as car batteries. Hydrofluoric acid is found in rust removers and tile cleaners. Hydrochloric acid is found in swimming pool cleaners and some toilet bowl cleaners, as well as the stomach's digestive juices. Common bases include sodium and potassium hydroxide, found in some drain and oven cleaners; sodium and calcium hypochlorite in household bleach; ammonia, in some cleaners and detergents; and phosphates in many household cleaners and detergents. Most of the household products are too dilute to cause serious contact burns to the skin. But they can cause severe damage to the eyes, and are very toxic if swallowed. Some of them can also give off dangerous fumes, especially if you mix ammonia and bleach, which produces chlorine gas.

Immediate treatment for a chemical burn is to remove the patient from the source and remove any contaminated clothing if you can do so without exposing yourself. Then continue flushing it with cool water for at least 15-20 minutes after the patient is no longer feeling a burning sensation, though if the chemical is in powder form, you should first brush it off before flushing. Flush each eye from the inner corner to the outside, so as to protect the tear duct and

the other eye. If both eyes are affected, you can position a nasal cannula over the bridge of the nose and connect it to a container of water or sterile saline so that it flushes from the inside corners outward.

Chemical fumes can irritate or damage the airways so that they swell, and inhaled chemical fumes can damage the lungs. So after any exposure to hazardous chemicals, you should monitor the airway and breathing, and administer oxygen if necessary.

Conclusion

Serious thermal burns can cause dehydration as well as damage to skin and underlying tissues, and partial thickness burns are among the most painful of injuries. Anyone who has been burned in a fire should also be assessed for inhalation injuries. In a wilderness or remote situation, after cooling the burn, you need to keep the patient warm and hydrated and (for an extensive burn) reduce fluid loss with occlusive dressings. Industrial electrical current passing through the body can cause much more damage than is apparent from the entrance and exit wounds, and affect breathing or heart function. So after making sure that the patient is no longer in contact with the source of electrical current, you may need to do basic life support. Many chemicals can cause burn-like injuries as well. Treatment is to brush away dry chemicals and flush wet chemicals with cool water.

Backpacking stoves: Function & safety

Fuels

All fuels produce carbon monoxide when they burn, so it is important for the cooking area to be well ventilated. Since carbon monoxide bonds very strongly to the hemoglobin in the blood, it reduces oxygen-carrying capacity for hours after exposure, so even if the dose is less than lethal, it reduces the body's ability to do work and generate heat, which increases the risk of both hypothermia and altitude illness.

Stove safety

Most backpacking stoves are only used occasionally. Tiny orifices can become clogged in storage, so test the stove before each trip. If your stove won't work, you will eat cold food, and in winter, be unable to melt snow for drinking water.

Stoves mounted on fuel tanks are tall with narrow bases, making them easy to upset along with a pot of hot food or water. Pot-and-windscreen kits widen a narrow stove's footprint, making it much safer.

A stove with a built-in tank can explode if wind shielding and the pot reflect too much heat into the tank.

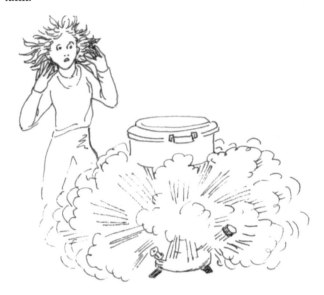

Cooking In tents

Many accidents can occur in tents, from trying to fill a tank before the stove has cooled or pouring fuel too near a flame. Stoves primed with liquid fuel frequently flare up when lit. The flare can burn a tent. Liquids boiling over or upset pots of boiling liquid can cause second or even third degree burns where people have no room to dodge.

Carbon monoxide poisoning is always a danger when cooking in a small enclosure (either a tent or a snow shelter). It has probably played a role in many deaths attributed to hypothermia.

Instant frostbite

Frostbite is an injury not usually associated with stoves and cooking. Yet liquid petroleum fuel escaping from pressurized canisters can cause frostbite in any weather if it strikes your skin, because it is chilled by expansion. Also, evaporation of liquid fuel on bare hands can quickly chill them below the freezing point of water in wind or cold weather. Spills are more likely if your hands are already numb from the cold. If you

pour fuel in cold weather, protect your hands by pulling thin rubber gloves over your glove liners.

Metal fuel bottles and canisters can also cause contact frostbite, if they've been out in the snow all night, and the fuel inside is chilled below the freezing point of water. So wrap them with duct tape, which also helps prevent dents and scratches that can weaken the fuel bottles.

Conclusion

Cooking with campfires requires dry firewood, which may not be available; and there are many restrictions on campfires in national parks and forests because of fire danger. So most campers carry stoves for cooking. No stove is absolutely safe or unsafe, under all conditions. To use stoves safely, know their hazards before you buy, and learn how to minimize the hazards when you are cooking. To pick the best stove for your activities, consider temperatures in the seasons when you will be camping, the size of your group, weight of stove and fuel, and whether your goal is to boil water rapidly or simmer gourmet meals.

Chapter 5. Bites, stings, and allergic reactions

Some blood sucking arthropods, like mosquitoes, use the protein from blood solids only to make eggs, which means that only the females bite. Others, like ticks, also live on blood. When they feed, these arthropods may transmit disease In the United States, ticks transmit over 99% of the disease that arthropods give to humans. Fleas carry plague, and in the tropics, other blood-sucking flies also carry diseases.

Worldwide, mosquitoes transmit the most disease to humans. In the United States, mosquito abatement programs in the first quarter of the 20th century reduced disease by reducing mosquito populations. However, there are more than enough mosquito vectors to cause epidemics in the United States, and we are protected from some tropical diseases only because no reservoirs (animal or human hosts carrying the disease) are available from which the mosquitoes can pick them up. Returning military personnel or immigrants infected with those diseases could change that. For example, some cases of malaria in a Girl Scout troop camping near the California coast were traced to an infected Vietnam veteran who was camping nearby.

Mosquitoes

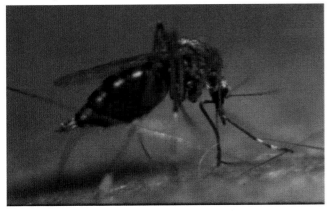

Mosquito feeding *Photo courtesy of Elton J. Hansons*

Mosquitoes need still or slow-moving water to breed, so they tend to be thickest in marshy terrain, and most abatement programs in the past depended on draining marshes, or killing the larvae with pesticides or oil at the cost of polluting the water. Mosquitoes can also breed in snowmelt pools, tree stump holes, ditches, or piles of used tires left outdoors. Most mosquitoes in the United States breed in spring and summer.

Mosquitoes sense hosts from a distance by odors. Midrange, carbon dioxide triggers a random flying reflex. If the flying brings the mosquitoes in close, heat and moisture attract them to the skin and trigger the blood-sucking reflex. The needle-like proboscis pierces the skin and injects blood-thinner with the saliva.

Protection

Repellents contain chemicals that interfere with the senses of bloodsuckers, making it hard for them to locate you. . For North American mosquitoes and other bloodsuckers, repellents with **DEET** (N-N-diethyl-meta toluamide) have been effective, though some species seem to become resistant to its effects after a few hours of exposure. DEET can eat holes in plastic and synthetic fabrics, so you should keep it away from clothing, packs, and tents. A 30% solution seems to be optimum. About 3% to 5% of the DEET applied is absorbed through the skin, and some studies suggest toxic effects. So it is probably best to minimize the amount of DEET that you put on your skin. One strategy is to use a mosquito shirt – a shirt made of mosquito netting that is kept in a bag saturated with DEET when you are not wearing it. Spraying clothing and mosquito netting with permethrin also helps.

Picaridin (brand name Bayrepel) is an alternative to DEET which seems to be at least as effective. It has much less odor than DEET, and does not damage plastic or synthetic clothing. Repellents with 30% **oil of lemon eucalyptus** (extracted from gum eucalyptus trees) have also scored well in *Consumer Reports* tests. Many other substances have some repellency, but are not very effective and do not last long on the skin.

Permethrin (which is sold under various brand names) attacks the nervous systems of arthropods on contact, usually causing them to drop off or fly away if it doesn't kill them. Permethrin is recommended only for spraying or soaking clothes and mosquito netting, not for use on the skin because it breaks down in contact with skin and can cause dermatitis. You should avoid inhaling it. Spray clothing outdoors while standing upwind. Once sprayed on clothing, it will stay active for weeks and for months in clothing that was soaked in a permethrin solution.. Be careful with permethrin treated clothing around pet cats or dogs, however, because they may rub against you, then ingest the permethrin by grooming themselves with their tongues; and ingested permethrin can cause liver damage.

Mosquito-borne diseases

Malaria is carried by an estimated 500,000,000 people, including more than half the population of Africa, and kills up to 1,200,000 per year according to a report published in *The Lancet* in 2012. About 90% of the deaths are in Africa. Although only about 1,000 cases of malaria are reported per year in the United States, almost all of them picked up in other countries, it is a serious threat to travelers in the tropics.

Malaria is caused by a **protozoan parasite**. *Plasmodium falciparum* and *P. vivax* cause most malaria infections, and *P. falciparum* causes 95% of the deaths, because it infects up to 60% of the red blood cells. *P. vivax* has only about 1% fatality, but is very debilitating. Also, *P. vivax* can remain in the liver for years after the host has apparently recovered, whereas when someone survives an infection by *P. falciparum*, the immune system usually clears out the parasite completely.

When the parasites swarm out of the liver into the blood, every third day, the patient experiences the symptoms of a malarial attack, which can last from one to eight hours. These symptoms include fever, shaking chills, sweats, headache, muscle pain and malaise. Victims of malaria also develop a palpably enlarged spleen, because one of its functions is to recycle worn out red blood cells.

The most recent remedy for P. falciparum infections, **artemisinin**, made from the leaves of *Artemesia annua* (sweet wormwood) trees, was discovered in an ancient Chinese herbal manual. Artemisinin combination therapy (ACT) combines several artemisinin derivatives with another anti-malarial drug. Since conditions and treatment may change rapidly, travelers should get the latest information about diseases in their destination countries from the website of the Centers for Disease Control and Prevention (www.cdc.gov).Travelers should also bring all necessary medications with them, because Africa and Asia are flooded with **counterfeit medications**.

The **yellow fever** epidemics in the United States from the 17th to the early 20th centuries were in seaports such as New Orleans, where travelers and sailors infected in the tropics provided a reservoir. It is caused by a virus, and transmitted mainly by *Aedes aegypti* and *A. albopictus* (Asian tiger) mosquitoes. Yellow fever infects about 200,000 people a year, with about 30,000 deaths, 90% in Africa and about 10% in South America. Early signs and symptoms, which can come on suddenly from three to six days after being infected, may include fever, chills, headache, muscle aches, nausea and vomiting. Jaundice – skin turning yellow – gives the disease its name. In more serious cases, the patient can also bleed from the nose and gums. A **vaccine** can provide protection for up to ten years, but there is no specific treatment.

Dengue fever is caused by a virus related to the yellow fever virus. Symptoms include fever, headache and pain behind the eyes, bone and joint pain (which is why it is also called breakbone fever). Dengue is a tropical disease, so most cases in the United States are brought back by travelers. Usually it lasts a week or less. But children can get a potentially fatal variation called dengue hemorrhagic ("bleeding") fever, which is an over-reaction of the body's immune system after they have started to recover from the virus. **Zika virus** (related to the Dengue virus) is common in Latin America and may spread to the United States.

Zika virus, which has been spreading through Latin America, is related to Dengue and transmitted by the same species of *Aedes* mosquitoes, so it could spread to North America. Symptoms are similar to those of Dengue, though three out of four victims may not realize they are infected because they have mild or no symptoms. Some researchers suspect that it can cause birth defects if a pregnant mother is infected.

Encephalitis means "inflammation of the brain," and mosquitoes transmit many viruses that infect the brain. No specific treatments or vaccines are available for any of them. Infections are rare in the U.S.

West Nile virus spread rapidly over the United States since 1999, when it was first reported, because its animal reservoir includes birds, and it is transmitted by 64 mosquito species. Symptoms may include fever, headache, nausea and vomiting. In 2015, 2175 cases (serious enough to require treatment) and 146 deaths in the U.S. were reported to the Centers for Disease

Control and Prevention (www.cdc.gov). About 80% of people infected, however, have no symptoms; and as with other infectious diseases, mild cases are often not reported, or even diagnosed, so West Nile virus infection is probably much more common than the statistics indicate.

Plague

Caused by bacteria (Yersinia pestis), this disease killed about one-third of the population in 14th century Europe. Since plague is carried by rodents, especially black rats, shipping routes have traditionally spread it from seaport to seaport. For millennia, when humans shared their houses with rats, they also shared the rats' fleas, which transmit the disease from host to host. Plague was probably introduced to the United States in San Francisco in 1899, and spread through the Western United States (as well as parts of Canada and Mexico) in wild rodent populations that live in burrows, including ground squirrels, deer mice, voles, and prairie dogs. So campgrounds are sometimes closed when infected rodents are found nesting in the grounds.

Only about ten human cases are reported per year in the United States. But infection is possible whenever a die-off of the wild rodent population leaves hungry fleas on their carcasses. Therefore, it is wise not to walk within flea-jumping distance (three feet or more) of a dead animal or to camp near rodent burrows.

Ticks

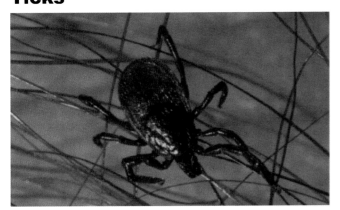

Tick on skin   *Photo courtesy of Jack C. Clark*

Soft ticks, which are found in burrows and nests, seldom contact humans and carry only one human disease - relapsing fever. Hard ticks are much more likely to find and feed on humans. Hard ticks wait for hosts in vegetation, and concentrate along animal trails and at boundaries (ecotones) where trails go from one type of vegetation to another (e.g., meadow to forest). Larvae and nymphs are usually in leaf litter, on the ground. Adults will wait on the tips of leaves or grass blades in the questing posture, holding on with their rear and middle legs and extending their forelegs.

Ticks have carbon dioxide sensors in their forelegs. Exhaled breath can stimulate the tick to drop onto a passing host or crawl up to 15 feet. At close range, heat and moisture trigger a reflex to grip and crawl upward on the host, against gravity. Then serrated mouthparts open the skin, and the barbed, hypostome ("under the mouth") secures the tick. Once attached, a hard tick will feed up to a week. An adult female can increase its weight a hundred-fold with a blood meal while regurgitating the liquid part of the blood back into the host and using the protein to make eggs. Larvae and nymphs also need blood meals to change to the next stage of their life cycle.

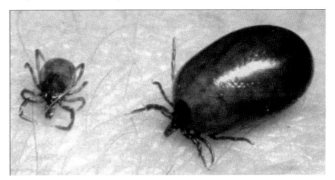

Ticks starting to feed (left) and swollen with a blood meal (right). *Photo courtesy of TickedOff.com*

Tick-borne diseases

Lyme disease is the best-known tick-borne infection and the most common - 300,000 cases per year in the U.S. estimated by the Centers for Disease Control and Prevention. In 1982, Willy Burgdorfer identified the corkscrew-shaped bacterium that causes Lyme disease, so it is named after him – *Borrelia burgdorferi*. It lives in the gut of an infected tick, and is stimulated to reproduce when the tick starts feeding. After a day or so, it crosses to the circulatory system and migrates to the salivary glands, where it can be injected into the host. But if the tick is properly removed before that, there is little chance of infection.

In the far Western United States, the tick that carries Lyme disease (*Ixodes pacificus*) has a low rate of infection, so there is little chance of catching Lyme disease from a single bite. But the tick that carries the disease in the Eastern United States (*Ixodes scapularis*) has a much higher rate of infection – 60% or more in parts of New England – because more of its animal hosts support the disease.

Lyme disease begins from 3 to 30 days after infection with flu-like symptoms, which may include chills and fever, fatigue, joint and muscle pain, and loss of appetite as the organism spreads through the blood stream. A rash around the bite, **erythema migrans** (spreading or "migrating redness"), appears in about 60% to 80% of infected adults and 90% of children.

Blood tests for Lyme disease are not completely reliable. The ELISA test can give a false positive for other infections; and the western blot test, given when the ELISA is positive or borderline, does not always detect Lyme disease. In 1998, a **vaccine** was licensed by Smith Kline Beecham, but withdrawn from the market in 2002.

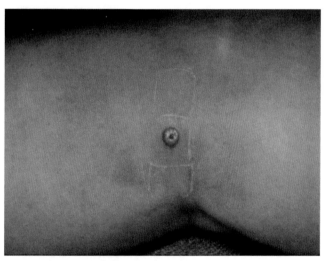

Rash of early stage Lyme disease (erythema migrans) surrounding the tick attachment site
Photo courtesy of Ben Schifrin, MD

In its early stages, Lyme disease can usually be cured with antibiotics. In its later stages, it may be more difficult to treat. If untreated, Lyme disease can persist for months or years. Signs and symptoms vary depending on where the bacteria go, possibly because there are many different strains of *Borrelia burgdorferi*. If they move to the synovial fluid of a joint, they cause arthritic symptoms, usually on just one side of the body - the most common form of late

stage Lyme disease in the United States. In the cerebrospinal fluid, the bacteria can cause neurological problems. In **Bell's palsy**, one or both sides of the face can be paralyzed for weeks to months.

Meningitis causes headache, a stiff neck, and light sensitivity. **Encephalitis** can cause sleeplessness, memory loss, and mood changes. Infection of the **heart** can cause arrhythmia, which usually clears up within weeks, but may require a pacemaker. If untreated, Lyme disease can become a chronic, recurring infection; but one possibility that may account for some seemingly intractable cases is that the patient had an undiagnosed co-infection from the tick.

If a tick has been feeding on you, and you experience the symptoms of Lyme disease within a month of the bite (whether or not you have a rash), you should have it treated with antibiotics.

If possible, bring back a tick alive in a ziplock bag containing damp paper toweling if it has fed on someone. A live tick can be tested in a Public Health Department for Lyme disease. Label the bag with the time and date that the tick was embedded and removed. Also note from what part of the body it was retrieved and the location where the tick was encountered.

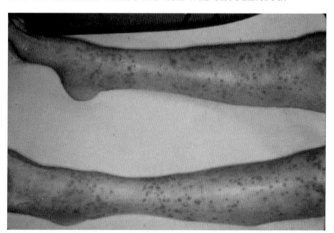

Rocky Mountain spotted fever
Photo courtesy of Ben Schifrin, MD

Rocky Mountain spotted fever was first recognized in the Bitterroot Valley of Montana, toward the end of the 19th century. Howard T. Ricketts correctly described it in 1910 as an infection carried by ticks. The organisms that cause this and many other diseases are named after him – *Rickettsiae*. They are very small bacteria that (unlike most bacteria) trick cells into ingesting them. Then they increase and multiply until the cells bursts. Since the spotted fever organisms infect cells in the walls of blood vessels, they cause many small hemorrhages. These hemorrhages show as spots on the skin and generally start on the limbs. But the real damage is inside vital organs.

Antibiotics can usually cure Rocky Mountain spotted fever if it is diagnosed and treated in time. Incubation ranges from two days to two weeks. The telltale spots may appear late (in 10% of cases) or not at all, so 2 - 3% of all victims still die, and 20% of those untreated or treated late. Fortunately, the infection rate in ticks that carry the disease is only 0.1%, but about 2,000 cases per year in the United States are reported to the Centers for Disease Control and Prevention each year, mostly in southern states.

Signs and symptoms may come on suddenly or after a few days of malaise. They often include a splitting headache and pains in the back, neck, joints, or legs. Light can become painful to the eyes, and a stiff neck can confuse the disease with meningitis. The victim is restless, sleeping poorly, often delirious, and runs a temperature of 104-106°, which is why it is called "fever."

Other Rickettsiae cause human **erlichiosis**, which afflicts several hundred people in the United States, mostly in the southeast and central states. Like Lyme disease, it has flu-like symptoms in the early stages: fever, chills, malaise, headache, and muscle pain. Later, the patient may suffer vomiting, coughing, abdominal pain, diarrhea, swollen lymph glands, and a rash. Erlichiosis can usually be cured with antibiotics.

Some ticks, including the one that carries Rocky Mountain spotted fever, can inject a toxin that causes a creeping **paralysis**. This paralysis starts in the hands and feet and moves up the limbs to the face. If it reaches the respiratory muscles, it can kill. In the United States, the paralysis is reversed by removing the tick, as the remaining toxin is cleared out of the system. But in Australia, there is a more potent tick toxin, whose effects continue after tick removal.

Tick protection and removal

Using repellents with DEET or picaridin on the skin and spraying or soaking clothes with permethrin, will help keep ticks off. Wear light-colored clothing so that you can see the dark brown ticks, and tuck your shirt into your pants. You should also wear long pants, tuck them into your socks, and wear gaiters. A hat saturated with permethrin will make it harder for ticks to get into your hair. Larvae and nymphs, and some adults, will be on the ground and crawl up your legs. Before feeding, adult Ixodes pacificus ticks are pinhead sized, and larvae and nymphs are barely visible specks.

Do frequent **tick searches** on yourself and your friends, especially before going into the tent for the night. Ticks that have crawled up the legs or body often seek warm, moist places to feed, such as the butt crack or armpit. Ticks that get onto the head when you brush against vegetation may be concealed under hair. A stiff back brush can help remove ticks crawling on your skin when you take a shower. To kill **ticks in clothing**, add borax or permethrin to laundry detergent, and use the hot setting for both washer and dryer.

There are several devices besides tweezers designed to remove ticks. The Tick Spoon is a small metal spoon with a V notch that you slide between the tick's body and embedded mouth parts to lever it out. The Tick Key has a keyhole shaped opening. Some devices come with a small magnifying glass to help you see what you are doing. Slowly pull the tick straight out and not twist, to avoid breaking off the body and leaving the mouthparts embedded. If the mouthparts remain embedded, however, remove them as you would a splinter.

Another method of tick removal is to use dental floss or strong thread. Tie a loose overhand knot, slip it over the tick, and gently close it around the tick as close to the skin as possible. Then slowly pull both ends of the floss or thread upward to remove the tick. Be careful not to touch the tick, since the Lyme disease organisms (which may have been released if the tick was damaged in removal) can penetrate unbroken skin.

None of the folklore techniques for removing ticks work. Anointing them with oil or nail polish won't kill them, because they can go for hours without breathing. Touching them with a hot match head won't do anything except possibly make them regurgitate, which could transmit any infection they may be carrying. If you remove the tick properly, however, you will reduce the chance of infection, even if the tick is carrying Lyme disease, because it takes about 24 hours after the tick attaches and starts feeding for the bacteria to migrate from the tick's gut to its salivary glands.

Venomous bugs

Venom may contain neurotoxin that paralyzes prey and enzymes that pre-digest prey before feeding. In humans, venom from bee, wasp, or ant stings usually just causes pain and swelling around the sting, though some spider venom is more potent. Victims who have been sensitized to venom by repeated exposure, however, may suffer an allergic reaction.

Bees and wasps usually attack only in defense of their nests or territories. While wasps can sting repeatedly, honeybees have a barbed stinger that usually cannot be retracted from human skin. The bee leaves the venom sack still pulsing and injecting venom as it pulls away. Scrape the sack off quickly with a credit card or whatever is handy.

Allergic reactions

Up to 4% of the United States population is allergic to stings, usually to bee, wasp, or ant venom. A local reaction will cause more pain and swelling spreading around the sting. A more widespread reaction is the eruption of red and itchy swellings over the body (hives). A full anaphylactic reaction can be fatal.

The word "anaphylaxis," from the Greek *an* (without) *phylaxis* (protection), is based on a misunderstanding. A researcher in 1913 was testing the effects of insect venom on dogs. He thought that the first dose of venom given to a dog had somehow knocked out the immune system, leaving the dog without protection against the second dose. In fact, the reverse happens. After repeated exposure, the immune system can over-react to the venom. Mast cells release histamines, which cause airways to constrict, swell, and congest, and blood vessels to dilate. The victim's face may swell alarmingly, and circulation will become sluggish as blood pressure drops.

The victim will be showing signs of respiratory distress, wheezing, and straining for breath. Treatment is **epinephrine** or an equivalent medication, which opens up the air passages.

Victims who know they are allergic may be carrying a bee-sting kit with an **epinephrine auto injector** (a hypodermic with a shielded needle that you just have to jab into a muscle). Another way to give the medication is with an epinephrine inhaler, if the victim still has enough airway open to suck in the aerosol.

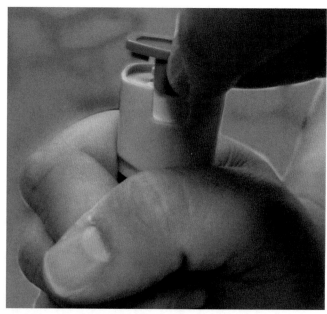

Remove the safety cap to release the needle.

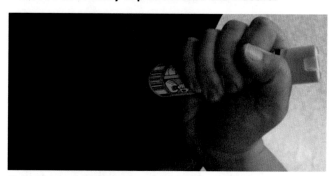

Grip the epipen firmly and jab it into the side of the thigh, midway between hip and knee, so that it goes into muscle. Hold for about 10 seconds. Do NOT put your thumb over the end, in case you have it reversed with the needle pointing outward. Document the time when you administered it.

An **antihistamine** will stop the mast cells from producing more histamines. The fastest route for the antihistamine is under the tongue. If the antihistamine is in a capsule, break the capsule open so that you can sprinkle the medication under the tongue for immediate absorption. You should also give oxygen if you have it.

Scorpions

As desert travelers know, scorpions are nocturnal feeders who seek shelter by day in crevices, or under wood or ground debris. They can also crawl into shoes, clothing, and sleeping bags, so it is important to shake these out before putting them on or crawling into them.

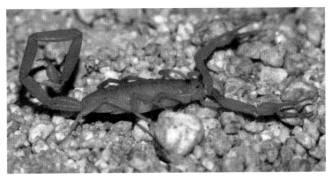

Arizona bark scorpion, Centrurodes sculpturatus.
Photo courtesy of Mike Cardwell

A mild scorpion envenomation causes pain and numbness around the sting site, and pain will increase if you tap on the site (tap test). If pain and numbness spread to other parts of the body, envenomation is more serious. In a severe case, the patient may have blurred vision, trouble swallowing, slurred speech, and upper airway problems. Restlessness or jerking and shaking of the extremities can mimic a seizure. Since 1968, however, no deaths have been reported from North American scorpions.

Treatment for scorpion stings is ice packs in cloth (30 minutes every hour) and oral pain killers. For stings with severe symptoms, the main concern is keeping the airway open and making sure that the patient is breathing normally. Doctors will usually give antivenom only if the symptoms are life-threatening, because it can cause an anaphylactic reaction.

Spiders

Most of the 30,000 species of spiders have venom glands, but only a few dozen species are dangerous to humans, because the others either do not have enough venom or can't penetrate human skin. The venom of hunting spiders has both neurotoxin to paralyze the prey, and digestive enzymes to liquefy the prey inside its husk so that the spider can suck it out. Neurotoxins can cause pain, and paralysis of muscles where the venom spreads.

Widow spiders

Widows are shy spiders found in sheltered corners of fields and gardens; under stones, logs, vegetation, wood piles; in wall crevices; and even in unoccupied buildings such as garages and barns. Widow spiders do not leave their webs, but defend them if disturbed.

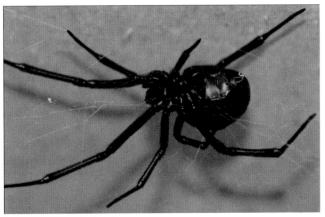

Female Western black widow spider
Photo courtesy of Mike Cardwell.

The females have bulbous bodies about 1 cm long, with a red hourglass marking on the abdomen. Their bite is usually painful from the start, though it may feel like a pinprick or cause a burning sensation. But within an hour, it will hurt more and more. Skin around the bite may sweat, and body hairs stand up. The neurotoxin causes neurotransmitter release, which can make muscles spasm and blood vessels constrict, increasing blood pressure (hypertension).

Other possible symptoms include abdominal, back or extremity pain; malaise; nausea and vomiting; headache; fever; or tremor. Respiratory muscle weakness may cause the victim to stop breathing. The victim usually recovers within days, but pain may continue for a week or more. In a pregnant woman, the venom can cause premature contractions. First aid includes cold packs for the pain, as well as cleaning the wound and checking tetanus immunization to prevent infection. There is a widow spider antivenom, but it is used only in cases of respiratory arrest, seizure, uncontrolled hypertension or pregnancy.

Recluse spiders

Loxosceles ("recluse") spiders are found worldwide in warm climates and are native to the southernmost United States. But they are also turning up in colder states as indoor spiders. They like warm, undisturbed environments such as vacant buildings, storage sheds, closets, and attics. They may nest in stored bed sheets or clothes. Recluse spiders are not aggressive, but may bite when threatened (e.g., when trapped against skin or shaken out of stored sheets). Females have slender bodies up to 1 cm long, and legs up to 3 cm long. They often have a dark, violin-shaped patch on top, so they are also called fiddle spiders.

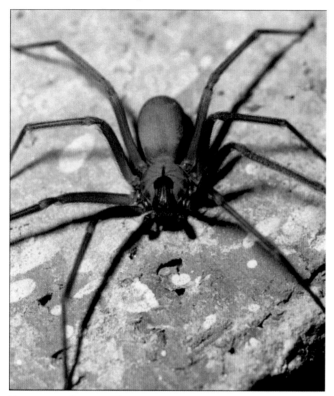

Brown recluse spider
Photo courtesy of Mike Cardwell

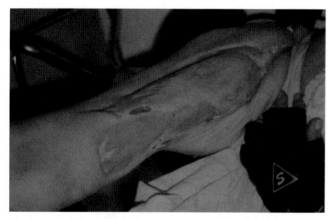

Recluse spider bite. *Photo courtesy Ben Schifrin, MD*

Their bite may be felt as a sharp stinging, or not be noticed. Also, if only a little venom is injected, it may cause only skin irritation. But moderate or severe envenomation causes serious tissue destruction. Severe envenomation may create an open, ulcerating wound, so make sure that tetanus immunization is up to date. Other possible effects of envenomation include swelling, elevated skin temperature, joint pain, malaise and nausea. Systemic effects, which are more frequent in children, may include blood in the urine, anemia, weakness, fever, and chills.

Other spiders

Many large, hairy spiders are called tarantulas because of the belief that their venom causes tarantism ("stupor and the desire to dance"). They are nocturnal hunting spiders with vertical fangs that rear back to strike, somewhat like rattlesnakes. Their bites are painful, but few species are dangerous. In fact, some of them are sold as pets.

The wandering spider (*Phoneutria nigrivin*) can travel with bananas exported from South America, so it is sometimes called the banana spider. Bananas may also have clusters of the wandering spider's eggs attached by spider silk, which look like small patches of white mold with dark spots. If venom is injected, it causes severe pain that radiates up. It can also cause sweating and salivation, nausea and vomiting, vertigo, visual disturbances, and priapism (uncontrolled erection). Victims usually recover in one to two days, though occasionally they die of respiratory paralysis. An antivenom is available in Brazil.

Snakebite

Africa, Asia, and Latin America have more species of venomous snakes with deadlier venom than North America; and much of their population still lives in rural areas where they are exposed to snakes. Estimates of fatal snakebites vary – possibly up to 100,000 per year in Asia, for example. But in the United States only 10 to 20 people per year die of snakebite.

Even though snakebite in the United States is seldom fatal, however, it can cause serious tissue damage. About 8,000 bites are reported every year, and probably many more go unreported. In 1927, almost all reported snakebites in the United States were accidental. Less than 5% were from intentional exposure to snakes and 59% were on the legs or feet. By 1988, 57% of the bites were from intentional exposure and 87% were on the arms or hands. Also, 28% of the victims were intoxicated.

Snakes of the United States

Venomous snakes usually bite humans only in defense, when surprised or threatened, because they can sense that we are too big for them to eat. They feed on small animals, especially rodents, and often play an important role in controlling rodent populations.

Rattlesnakes, cottonmouths, and copperheads account for 98% of human bites in the U.S. The other 2% of bites are from coral snakes, and from foreign snakes in zoos or kept as pets. Cottonmouths are similar to rattlesnakes, but they are found mainly in swampy areas of southern states.

Rattlesnakes, cottonmouths, and copperheads are called pit vipers because they have heat-sensing pits behind the nostrils that guide their strike at the warm prey. Their sense of smell is augmented when the forked tongue picks up odor molecules from the air and brings them to receptors in the roof of the mouth. They have slit pupils, which can admit more light to adapt them for night hunting. Their eyes are sensitive to motion, but cannot focus sharply because they have no fovea. They also lack external ears, but they can sense ground vibration with the middle ears.

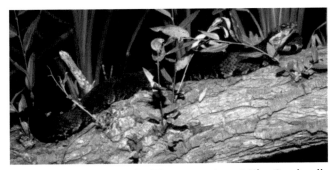

Western cottonmouth. *Photo courtesy Mike Cardwell*

Copperheads are found in central and southeastern states but their bite, though painful, is not very dangerous. Most serious snakebites in the United States, therefore, come from rattlesnakes, which are found in every contiguous state except Maine.

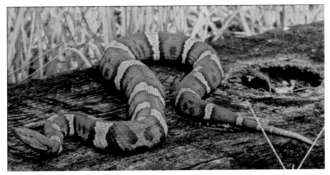

Trans Pecos Copperhead. Photo courtesy of Mike Cardwell

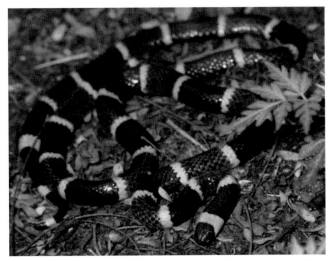

Texas Coral snake. *Photo courtesy of Mike Cardwell*

Coral snakes, found only in the South and Southwest of the U.S., are small, shy snakes with small mouths, and chew to inject venom. So they account for less than 1% of venomous bites in the U.S., almost all to people handling the snakes. But their venom is a potent neurotoxin, which can paralyze and even kill from respiratory or heart failure. U.S. species have narrow yellow bands between the red and black bands.

Rattlesnake habitats and behavior

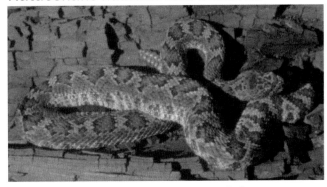

Rattlesnake. *Photo courtesy of Ben Schifrin, MD*

Most forest is too cool for rattlesnakes, but they are found in brushy or rocky hills, grassy meadows, and desert. In the mountains, they may be found up to 9,000 feet and up to 11,000 feet in the California summer. Since they have no sweat glands or internal temperature regulation, the temperature range in which they can function is limited. Rattlesnakes are most active at 80-90° F. Below 61° F, they seek shelter, and at 46° F they are immobilized.

When the temperature drops, they may coil up on a rock or an asphalt road that is radiating heat. On a warm night, however, they are likely to be out hunting.

They hibernate in winter and are most active in spring because they are hungry after hibernation, and it is mating season. Rattlesnakes do most of their growing in the first two years but can live up to 30 years.

In response to a threat, rattlesnakes may freeze and blend into the surroundings, or retreat (sometimes keeping their heads raised and poised to strike). When cornered, they may go into a striking coil but they can strike from any position, especially if handled.

Fangs and venom

When a rattlesnake strikes, the mouth opens 180°, aiming the fangs at the prey. The venom glands and ducts are contracted by the external jaw muscle, independently of the striking and biting action; and the size of the prey or threat (gauged by the heat-sensing pits) determines the amount of venom injected.

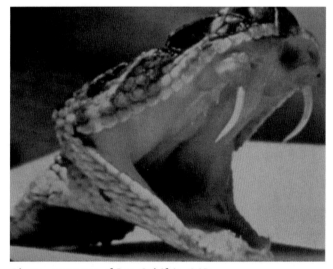

Photo courtesy of Ben Schifrin, MD

In humans, a mature snake may inject 25% to 75% of its venom. A glancing angle or protective clothing may prevent enough penetration to inject venom. About 20% of rattlesnake bites are dry, with no venom injected, and about 30% inject only a little venom. The remaining 50% of bites inject enough venom to cause moderate to severe damage in humans. Baby rattlesnakes also have venom, so they are dangerous even though they do not have the striking range and power of mature snakes.

Rattlesnake venom immobilizes and then kills prey; predigests the prey inside its skin. Peptides in the venom kill prey by damaging cell membranes and the walls of blood vessels, causing fluid loss and shock. In humans, the dose is almost never enough to kill,

though the enzymes can cause swelling, blisters, and serious tissue destruction.

Venom of rattlesnakes or other pit vipers can also cause long-term impairment of function, especially in people bitten on a hand or finger. Some components of the venom can cause leakage of red blood cells and fluid shifts from the blood, lowering the blood pressure (hypotension). Neurotoxins, which paralyze prey, can cause numbness and partial paralysis in humans. Some Mojave rattlesnake venom has especially potent neurotoxins, which can occasionally paralyze the breathing muscles in humans.

Weakness, numbness (usually around the scalp, face and lips) and nausea occur in about three-fourth of rattlesnake bite victims as the venom spreads. Pain and swelling start within minutes, and with severe envenomation, can spread to the whole limb in one hour. Usually, if no pain or swelling occurs after 20 minutes, either the bite was dry or it was not a rattlesnake. About one-fourth of victims develop blood blisters from 6 to 36 hours after the bite, which spread up the limb.

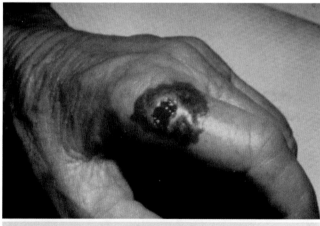

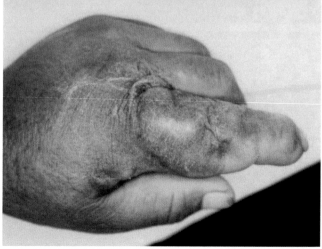

Rattlesnake bite: Progressive swelling and blistering
Photos courtesy of "Ben Schifrin, MD.

Treatment

The infamous snakebite kits with razor blades have probably done more damage than snakes. Slashing, especially around the hands, wrists and ankles (which are commonly bitten), can cut nerves and tendons as well as blood vessels. Trying to suck venom out with the mouth can infect the bite, and ice will not help.

For the bites of snakes whose venom is likely to be fatal if it spreads to the heart and other vital organs, such as cobras, bushmasters, and mambas, use an elastic bandage to immobilize and compress the entire area over and around the bite, or the entire limb if the bite is to an arm or leg. This will slow the spread of the venom by shutting down the lymph system, allowing more time to reach a hospital with the appropriate antivenom. In North America, however, only coral snake bites (or bites from deadly exotic snakes bought as pets) require the pressure bandage treatment.

For rattlesnake and other pit viper bites, there is no evidence that a pressure bandage would be helpful, and it might increase local tissue damage. Constricting bands are not helpful either, especially if they are too tight, and act like a tourniquet.

If the bite is to the hand or arm, it may help to immobilize the arm loosely and keep it below the heart. Plastic suction pumps are advertised for removing venom, but no published studies support their use, and a recent study done on pigs showed no significant venom extraction or effect on swelling.

Keeping the patient calm and limiting physical activity may help to slow the spread of venom. Drinking fluids will help to prevent shock. If no pain or swelling occurs within 20 minutes, however, and no other signs or symptoms are found, then probably no venom was injected.

Once you have done the first aid, you should get the patient as quickly as possible to a hospital that has antivenom. Call ahead to the hospital because they will have to order antivenom sent by air if it is not stocked. Also, describe the effects of the venom (e.g., the hand is swollen to twice its normal size), so that they will believe you. During evacuation, mark the boundary of the swelling and the time on the patient's skin every 15 minutes with a sharpie pen, to provide a graphic record of the venom's progressive effects.

Antivenom is the same for all pit vipers. It won't prevent tissue damage, unless it is administered within 30 minutes of the bite; but if administered within 24 hours of the bite it can reverse systemic effects such as hypotension, coagulopathy (blood doesn't clot), nausea, and loss of nerve function. But it costs the hospital over $2000 per vial - a fraction of what the hospital will bill the patient.

Bears and other mammals

In the United States, there are an average of just two injuries and one death per year from bear attacks. Why are there so few bear attacks on humans? Probably because for centuries bears that showed aggression toward humans were killed and eliminated from the gene pool. By contrast, deer kill dozens of people every year by jumping in front of speeding cars. So driving cautiously and watching for deer on back country roads is more likely to save your life on a wilderness trip than a 44 magnum or a can of pepper spray.

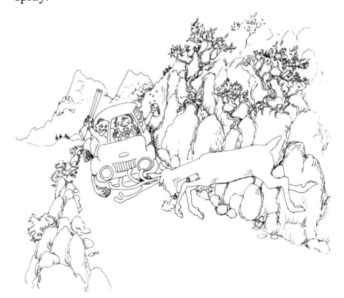

In popular wilderness areas, bears have become habituated to humans and associate them with food. So store food (and anything that smells of food) well away from camp sites. In a wooded area, one technique is to hang the food between two trees with 1/8" braided nylon cord (too thin to chew) and secure the ends of the cord around two other trees further away.

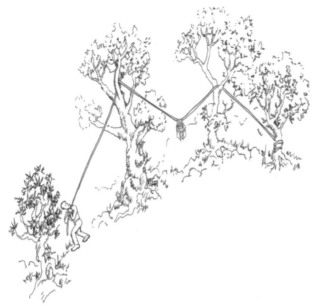

To avoid close encounters with bears, make plenty of noise when hiking through their territory, so as not to blunder into them when the wind does not carry your scent to them. When confronted with an aggressive bear, it is usually best to back slowly away while avoiding the challenge of eye contact; but never run because that can trigger predator-prey behavior, and bears can sprint faster than humans.

Rabies and hantavirus

Rabies is caused by a virus transmitted in saliva, usually by bites, but sometimes by aerosol in bat caves where saliva rains down from clusters of bats on the roof. Besides dogs and bats, it is also carried by skunks, raccoons, cats, monkeys (especially in Asia), foxes, and wolves. In the United States, the disease kills only a few people each year, because it has been almost wiped out in domestic dogs by vaccination and quarantine. But in countries with a high risk of rabies, such as India, you should know where the nearest source of modern vaccine is. Given after exposure, but during the incubation period (before the virus attacks the nervous system) the best vaccine is 100% effective.

Hantavirus, found in most Western states, is usually transmitted by inhaling the dust from dried deer mouse droppings when cleaning cabins. Early signs and symptoms are vague: fever, chills and muscle aches within three to five days. Victims may later suffer headache, nausea, vomiting, abdominal pain, diarrhea and cough. To clean rodent droppings safely

where hantavirus has been reported, wet them with bleach, and wear a respirator and rubber gloves.

Marine hazards

Bacteria that can cause wound infections thrive in the saline medium of the oceans, and are also common in fresh water. The teeth or spines of marine animals that inflict wounds are also usually contaminated with dangerous bacteria. So any wound inflicted in water is likely to become infected, especially if there are foreign bodies or venom in it. It is therefore especially important to clean marine wounds thoroughly by irrigating with fresh water and removing any foreign matter that does not flush out. Most marine injuries, however, are from encounters with organisms that have stinging cells (such as jellyfish) or spines (such as sea urchins or stingrays). Attacks on humans by large predators such as sharks are rare.

If stung by a **jellyfish** or anemone, remove any adhering jellyfish tentacles or stinging cells with a paste of baking soda, sand or mud and seawater, and scrape them off. Do NOT use fresh water or urine because it will trigger any unfired stinging cells on the skin. Soak the skin with vinegar, which inactivates any stinging cells on the skin that have not yet fired. Then monitor the patient for allergic reactions.

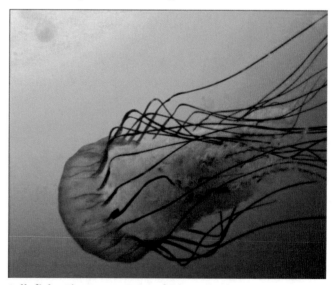

Jellyfish. *Photo courtesy of Oleg Grachev*

Stingrays are flat bottom dwellers in warm water shallows that often lie buried in the sand except for their eyes and spiracles. Species range in size from a few inches across to 12 feet by 6 feet. They are the most common cause of fish envenomation, with an estimated 2,000 stinging injuries per year in the United States. Usually the victim was walking in the surf during the spawning season and stepped on the stingray. Its whip-like tail, which has one or more barbed stingers, snaps forward and drives the spike into the victim. To avoid this reaction, scuff your feet in the sand when walking through surf in stingray breeding season, so as to warn them of your approach.

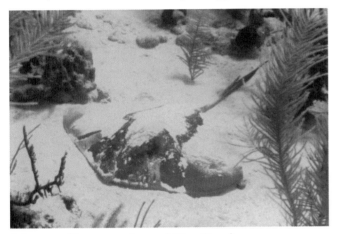

Stingray. *Photo courtesy of Oleg Grachev*

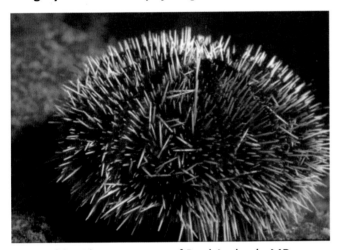

Sea urchin. *Photo courtesy of Paul Aerbach, MD*

Sea urchins are slow moving invertebrates with hollow spines that (in some species) are venomous. Most injuries are to people wading in tidal pools or beaches who step on or handle a sea urchin. Symptoms of severe envenomation may include muscle aches and weakness, breathing problems, and paralysis. Spines may break off in the skin – remove them with tweezers. Starfish have similar spines. To treat envenomation by stingray, sea urchin, or starfish immerse the spiked extremity in hot water (as hot and as long as you can tolerate). This will help inactivate the venom.

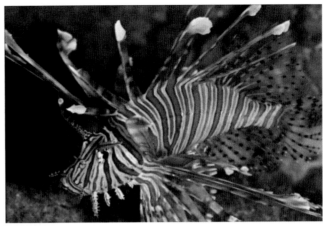

Lionfish. *Photo courtesy of Oleg Grachev*

Lionfish, native to the Indian Ocean, are now found on the East Coast and in the Caribbean, in lagoons, coral reefs, and rocky surfaces. They are small but aggressive fish with venomous spines.

Catfish also have spines that can inflict stings. Perhaps the strangest of them is the Amazonian Candiru ("urethra fish"), which is just 1" long and transparent. It can swim into the urethra of someone urinating in the water and lock itself in place by extending its spines. Mega-doses of vitamin C may help to dislodge it. Normally it is a parasite that swims into the gill slits of fish (against the current of the water being forced out) and attaches itself.

Sea snakes are not aggressive and have very small mouths, so human envenomation is rare, and usually from snakes caught in fishing nets. In about 75% of sea snake bites, there is no envenomation. But because the venom is so deadly, get the patient to a hospital that has or can get the antivenom – call ahead in case they have to send for it. Meanwhile, wrap the entire limb in an elastic bandage, so as to slow the spread of venom through the lymph system, as with any other potentially deadly snake venom.

Hazardous plants
Leaves of Three

Three plants in the United States are the most notorious for causing allergic reactions: poison oak, poison ivy and poison sumac. Poison oak grows as a low shrub in the East and South but is found as both a tall shrub and a clinging vine on the Pacific Coast. Poison ivy has many varieties and can grow as a shrub as well as a vine. It is found in wooded areas, and near lakes and streams through most of the United States, though not in the Pacific Coast states. Poison sumac grows as a shrub in swampy areas of the Eastern states. Poison oak and ivy leaves usually grow in clusters of three – poison sumac has clusters of 12 leaves or more.

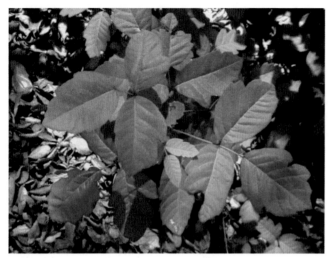

Poison Oak. *Photo courtesy of Linda Garcia*

All of them have an oil called urushiol ("milky oil") in their sap, to which many people are allergic. When the plants are in leaf, you can pick up the oil by brushing against them, because the black, sticky sap can accumulate on the surface. But urushiol is also in the plants' stems and roots. It can seep through contaminated clothing to skin. It can rapidly penetrate the skin and combine with skin proteins, so to get it all off you would need to remove it within 10 or 15 minutes. Dogs can romp in the plants and bring back uroshiol on their fur. Free ranging pet cats that sleep with you or curl up with you on the sofa can spread it over your whole body. If the plant burns, the oil can be inhaled in smoke, which sometimes kills forest fire fighters.

A cool shower with strong soap (before the oil is absorbed through the skin) should get most of it off, though several products are specially designed to remove urushiol, such as Tecnu Poison Oak and Ivy Cleanser®. You should make sure that no leaves or twigs are still in your clothes or equipment, and isolate clothes that may be contaminated for a separate wash with detergent and Tecnu. Calamine lotion or a tepid bath with baking soda may relieve some of the itching. For a severe reaction with swelling, a doctor can prescribe a steroid, like prednisone. Topical steroid creams and antihistamines usually have little effect.

Plants that sting or stab

Some plants have stinging hairs on their leaves that can inject irritating substances if you brush against them. In the United States, the most common ones are stinging nettles and spurge nettles. Soaks and cold compresses may relieve the itching.

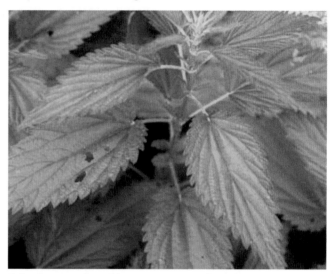

Stinging nettles. *Photo courtesy of Linda Garcia.*

Cactuses have spines that may be almost invisibly small, as in the prickly pear, or large enough to cause serious wounds.

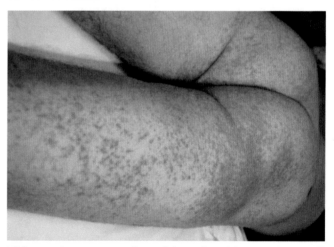

This patient was pincushioned with many small cactus needles.

One way to remove tiny hair-like spines is to lay sticky tape over them and peel it off. You can also coat the area with rubber cement and let it dry before peeling. Always peel in the direction that body hairs are oriented. Lift up the edge of the dried coating with your fingernails to start it.

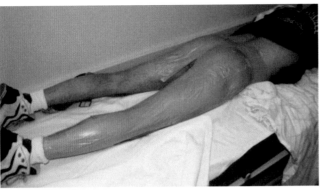

Needles removed by covering with tape, then peeling it off. *Photos courtesy of Ben Schifrin, MD*

Large cactus spines that have penetrated deeply may have to be removed surgically, which can be difficult because they may break off under the skin, and they do not always show on x-rays.

Conclusion

Blood sucking bugs can transmit diseases, so it is important to protect yourself against them by using repellants and clothing treated with permethrin. Stings by venomous bugs can cause allergic reactions, which can be life-threatening unless the patient is carrying medication that opens the constricted airway. Venomous snakes usually attack humans only in defense. Bears and other wild mammals kill or injure very few people in the United States, but they have learned to associate people with food; so safe storage of food in the wilderness will help to avoid close encounters. Keeping your distance from any wild mammal is also important for avoiding diseases they may be carrying, such as rabies or plague (in infected fleas). Large marine predators seldom attack humans, but many smaller marine organisms have defensive stinging cells or spines that can inflict painful injuries. Some plants also have potentially painful defenses. So we need to be able to identify and avoid biological hazards in the wilderness, and treat injuries they may cause. We also need to avoid popular treatments that can do more harm to the patient than the original injury.

Chapter 6. Bone and Joint Injuries

In an adult, bone is about two-thirds mineral and one-third tough protein fiber, a composite that combines density and rigidity with resistance to bending stress. Children's bones have less mineral and more protein fiber, which makes their bones more flexible and less likely to break. They also have growth plates at the ends of their long bones, however, and injury to these plates can stunt growth of the bone.

Under a magnifying glass, a cross-section of bone shows a honeycomb structure, with material following lines of stress. Red blood cells are made in the spaces of this honeycomb at the ends of long bones, and in the ribs and vertebrae. Each bone is enclosed by a membrane called the periosteum ("around the bone") containing nerves and blood vessels that penetrate the bone through a network of canals. So cracked or broken bones bleed, and broken bone ends can cause more bleeding by cutting blood vessels. Fractures also hurt and continue to hurt, though the pain may be masked for a while by the epinephrine rush of an athletic activity. Finger pressure on the fracture causes a sharp, local pain (point tenderness), which helps distinguish the injury from the diffuse pain of a bruise.

Keeping bone Strong

Many elderly people are vulnerable to fractures because they have osteoporosis ("porous bone"). They have lost so much bone mass and mineral content that the honeycomb structure is mostly air. These fragile bones can break even before the victim hits the ground. Women past menopause are especially vulnerable to osteoporosis.

To prevent osteoporosis, you need to do regular weight and stress-bearing exercise to stimulate the replacement of calcium. Bone responds (within limits) to the demands that you put on it. Thus as you get older, your choice is to use it or lose it. Running and other sports that weight and impact the leg bones will help maintain their bone mass and density, but do little for the upper body. Weight lifters generally have the strongest, densest bones, and even elderly people have regained some lost bone mass by regular resistance exercise, providing that they increased the weight as they grew stronger.

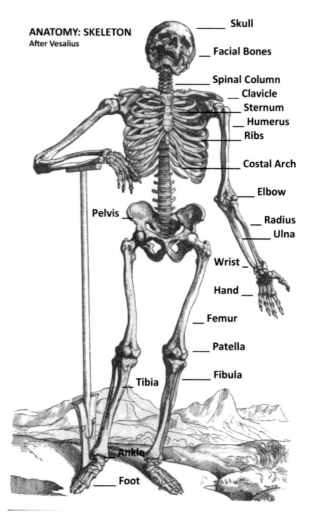

ANATOMY: SKELETON
After Vesalius

- Skull
- Facial Bones
- Spinal Column
- Clavicle
- Sternum
- Humerus
- Ribs
- Costal Arch
- Elbow
- Radius
- Ulna
- Pelvis
- Wrist
- Hand
- Femur
- Patella
- Fibula
- Tibia
- Ankle
- Foot

Mechanisms of bone Injury

Bone can be damaged by many mechanisms of injury, and reconstructing the mechanism will give clues to the damage. A direct blow from a fall, collision or the impact of a fast-moving object can crack a bone or break it completely. A crushing blow can shatter bone into fragments. An indirect blow radiating up an extended arm or stiffened legs can injure any bone or joint in the limb and beyond. A bending force, caused for example by a ski wedged in heavy snow or a foot jammed between rocks as the body continues to move, can snap a bone. A slow twisting fall on skis, when the bindings do not release, can break the bone in a spiral pattern. Repetitive impact stress from backpacking or running can cause a hairline or displaced fracture in the foot.

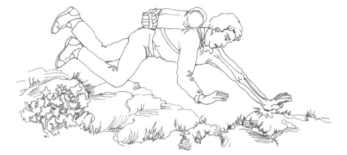

The victim of a fracture may have heard something crack, and if spasming muscles are moving broken bone ends against each other, you may hear a faint grating sound (crepitis). The patient will probably be guarding the injured bone – cradling it or at least unwilling to move it.

Assessing bone injuries

The pain of a fracture can mask other injuries, so you should do a quick assessment of the whole body after acknowledging and looking at the injury that is the patient's chief complaint. As you do the assessment, visualize the mechanism of injury and ask yourself what other injuries are likely from the same mechanism (**associated injuries**). Also check for injuries common to the type of accident.

When checking the injured limb, first ask where it hurts and work around that area to check the rest of the limb. Also remember to check functions distal to the injury, as described in the chapter on patient assessment: circulation, sensation, movement (CSM).

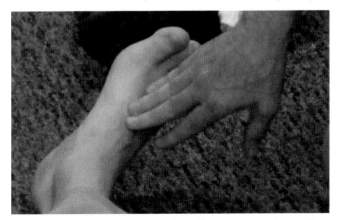

Dorsalis pedis ("top of the foot") pulse: just lateral to the tendon that enables you to raise the big toe.

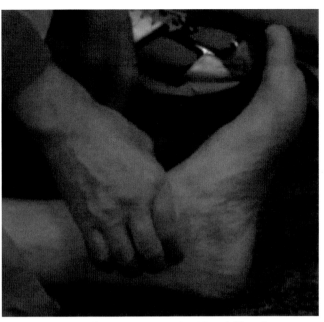

Posterior tibial ("behind the tibial knob") pulse.
Photos courtesy of Lynn Garcia.

This is important because a fracture can crimp or damage an artery or nerve. If any distal functions are impaired (weaker than on the uninjured limb) or absent, you should apply gentle inline tension to the fractured bone then check again. Grip the limb near the joints and gently stretch it out. After splinting, re-check distal functions to ensure that the splint is not impairing circulation or nerve function.

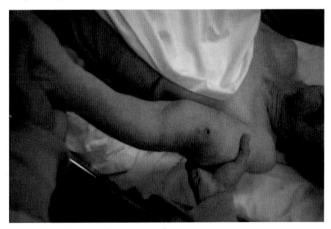

Angulated open humerus fracture.
Photo courtesy of Ben Schifrin, MD

What signs would suggest a fracture?
Deformity
- A fractured limb may be bent out of line at the break, making an angle.

- If the broken bone ends are shifted sideways, you may see a step deformity.
- If the muscles spasm, they may move the broken bone ends like an extra joint (false motion).

Rotation

- In a hip fracture, the leg and foot are usually rotated outward. A spiral fracture of the lower leg from a twisting fall could also rotate the foot.

Shortened limb

- The bone may be impacted, which means driven into itself or its socket by an impact on the extended limb.
- In a femur fracture, spasming muscles can also shorten the limb by driving broken bone ends past each other into the soft tissues.

Tenting

- You may see tenting – a broken bone end pushing up under the skin – or blood under the skin.

As you feel a limb, you are checking for point tenderness as well as deformity, so you need to grip with both hands and feel every inch.

Keep one eye on the patient's face and back off if you get an "Ouch!" Otherwise, you should grip firmly enough to feel the bone. Some bones, such as the femur, are sheathed in thick layers of muscle, but other bones are more accessible. For example, you can feel most of the humerus on the outside of the upper arm and the tibia (shinbone) on the front of the lower leg.

When checking a fracture in the upper arm (humerus), have the patient make a fist and then extend the fingers of the injured arm. If the patient can do this, then the radial nerve, which wraps around the humerus, is intact. Touching the tip of the thumb to the base of the little finger tests the median nerve. And spreading the fingers into a fan tests the ulnar nerve. Given this information, an orthopedist may not need to operate to repair a nerve, even if the patient develops wrist drop later because swelling is compressing the radial nerve.

Open and closed fractures

Any fracture that has a deep open wound near it has an open pathway for infection all the way to the bone marrow, even if the bone is not sticking out. So the first problem is to treat the wound. If serious bleeding occurs, you may not be able to put much direct pressure on it, so you might need to use a tourniquet. If

bleeding is not a problem, then you need to irrigate and protect the wound first, then position the splint so it does not put pressure on the wound. A closed fracture is still enclosed by the skin and underlying tissues. One goal of treatment is to keep it that way and not turn it into an open fracture by mishandling the limb.

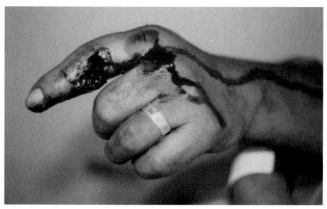

Open finger fracture. *Photo: Ben Schifrin, MD*

Principles of splinting

Not only does a fracture bleed and hurt; the broken bone ends can cause further damage to the soft tissues around them as the limb moves or the muscles spasm. To prevent this damage, you need to immobilize the broken bone ends. Since muscle attachments go across joints, you also need to immobilize the joints adjacent to a fracture. Otherwise the muscles contracting to move those joints could also move those broken bone ends. After splinting a fractured limb, you should elevate it if possible to reduce swelling.

A splint is anything that immobilizes the injured bone and adjacent joints. Narrow boards or stiff cardboard are traditional splints for urban first aid, though a magazine wrapped around the limb or anything else that gives support can do the job. In the wilderness, if you are not carrying a ready-made splint, you can improvise with a stick, tent pole, ice ax, a metal stave from an internal frame pack, a foam pad, or any other materials at hand.

Pad a hard splint:
- To fill any empty space between the splint and the limb, e.g. at the wrist, providing firm and even support along the whole length of the limb;
- To prevent pressure damage to the skin and to nerves that pass over bone close to the skin;
- To insulate a metal splint.

Think about which bones you are trying to immobilize and where they lie when you are positioning the splint. For example, to splint the forearm a hard splint should usually be on the palm side, so that it will be closest to both bones and can support the hand in a relaxed position. To secure a splint to the limb, you can use cravat bandages, cloth ties, gauze roller bandages, surgical wrap, tape, or anything else that is wide enough to distribute the pressure over the limb, and not cut off circulation.

You can wrap a stretchy bandage the whole length of the splint, adjusting the tension for the patient's comfort; but avoid putting ties directly over the break. To immobilize a broken bone end, a non-stretchy tie should be a few inches from the break so that it does not press on the break, but close enough to apply maximum leverage and immobilize the bone end. Put the knots on the outside of the splint, where you can reach them if you need to adjust the tension.

For a forearm splint, the hand should be in the position of function - the relaxed position that equalizes muscle tension on both sides. If you hold your forearm up vertically and relax the hand, you will see that the wrist is slightly extended (bent back) and the fingers half curled. Place a roller or a wad of padding under the palm, or let the fingers curl around the end of the splint. In a leg splint, the knee should be slightly flexed, not hyperextended.

Handling a fractured limb

Before you start to splint, organize and lay out your equipment, so that once you begin you can continue without interruption until the limb is secured. An assistant or the patient can stabilize the injured limb or hold the splint in place as you are securing it to avoid jiggling. If you are splinting a leg and the patient is on the ground, you can usually get ties into place without moving the limb - just slide them under the spaces behind the knee or ankle and into place.

If you need to move a fractured limb to get the ties or splint in place, you should support it so that you will not put a bending stress on the fracture. If the patient has long pants or sleeves, have your partner gather up the slack of the cloth in both hands, on either side of the fracture, so that the clothing is snugly wrapping the limb, and then lift. If you are working

alone, slide a stick or pole inside the pant leg and then grip the cloth around the stick to lift the leg.

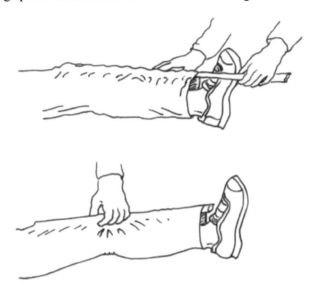

Another way is to grip the limb near the joints and apply gentle inline tension (pulling apart) to prevent the break from sagging as you lift. But you should never just pick up an unsplinted, fractured limb by one or even both ends, because the fracture could sag, causing pain and possible further damage. While you lift the limb, your partner can put the splint in position.

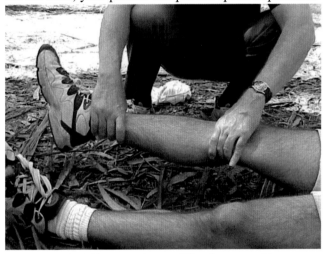

Using gentle inline tension to lift a fractured leg
Photo courtesy of Ruth McConnell

Types of ready-made splints

Large groups that do not have to carry everything on their backs (e.g., river rafting trips) may carry **air splints**. These are double-walled sleeves of transparent plastic that you fit over the injured limb and inflate until they apply enough pressure to immobilize the limb without impairing circulation.

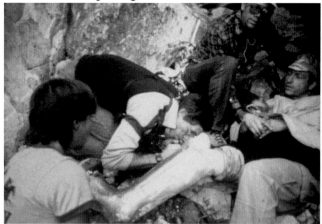

Photo courtesy of Ben Schifrin, MD

Their advantages are that they can be applied quickly, reduce swelling by putting pressure on the entire limb, and are transparent, so you can check the appearance of the limb. Their disadvantages are that they are heavy and expensive, they can leak, they trap perspiration and stick to the skin, and if you are gaining or losing altitude, you need to adjust the pressure.

Photos courtesy of SAM Medical Products

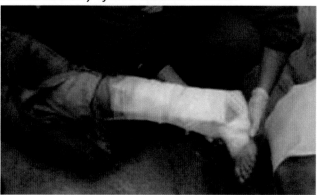

SAM splint wrapped around both sides of the lower leg to stabilize a fracture

SAM splints (www.sammedical.com), developed by Dr. Sam Scheinberg, are much lighter and more versatile alternatives and are carried by many ski patrollers and wilderness rescuers. They are made from a thin sheet of aluminum padded with foam on both sides, 4" by 36," can be folded up or rolled for carrying and weigh just 4 oz. They are also radio-lucent, so they don't have to be removed for x-rays. You bend the splint into a half-cylinder to give it strength, then mold

it to the uninjured limb to get an exact fit before applying it to the injured arm or leg. You can use it double thickness to make an extra strong splint, or fold it into a sugar tong so that it wraps both sides of a limb (as in the two SAM splint photos).

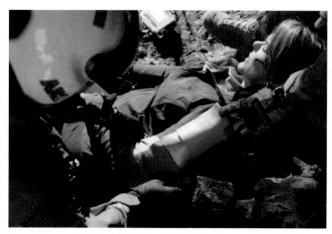

Applying a SAM splint to stabilize a humerus fracture

You can combine two SAM splints to make an extra-long sugar tong splint for the leg. You can also shape the SAM splint into a rigid triangle to support a locked knee or a dislocated shoulder that is locked in an awkward position. SAM splints have illustrated directions printed on them, and instructional videos can be downloaded from their web site.

Soft Splints

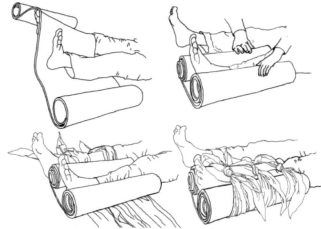

For a fractured lower leg or ankle, a foam sleeping pad makes an excellent splint. Lift the leg, using one of the techniques already described, and slide the foam pad underneath so about half of the length is on either side of the leg. Then roll up the pad on either side until the two rolls are snug against the leg. If you are working alone, kneel below the patient's feet and clamp the two rolls against the leg with your knees. Slide two or three cravats or other ties into position under the pad and fasten them with the knots in accessible positions.

A blanket or bulky garment can make a good splint for an injured ankle. In cold weather, you could leave the boot or shoe on for warmth and additional support, but loosen the laces and check regularly to make sure that swelling is not impairing circulation or nerve function. Fold the blanket or jacket into a rectangle about 1' x 3'. If the patient is sitting or lying on the ground, slide three cravat bandages under the ankle, slipping them through the space behind the Achilles tendon. Then fold the blanket around the bottom of the foot so that it wraps the ankle and lower leg on both sides. Now slide one cravat up almost to the upper edges of the blanket and tie it, pulling it as tight as is comfortable for the patient. Tie the second cravat around the ankle.

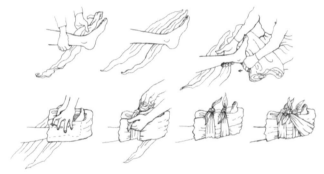

Spread out the third cravat so that it cups the bottom corner of the blanket, bring it diagonally to the instep and tighten it as much as the patient will tolerate. This tie really snugs up the splint. If you are using a rolled up jacket instead of a blanket, and it does not give enough support, add a figure 8 bandage: loop the center of a cravat around the booted toes, cross the tails, pass them around the splint and under the ankle, bring them back up and tie them.

The swivel hitch

If you are improvising a splint with sticks or poles, the swivel hitch is a helpful technique. If you just wrap ties around both the stick and the much thicker limb, the stick can slide around within the wrap. If a fractured leg is already on the ground in a good position, you can usually apply a splint without moving the leg.

Start by sliding the ties in place under the leg. For a supine patient, use the spaces behind the knee and Achilles tendon, then slide the ties into position. Leave about 2/3 of each tie on the outside. You can use a single stick or pole (on the outside), or one on each side. Then slide the stick(s) or pole(s) under the ties, next to the leg, and wrap each tie around the stick(s). Put padding in place, e.g., a spare jacket draped over the leg so that it will hang down between the leg and the stick(s). Then bring both ties across the leg, bring the outer tie under and around splint and leg again, tighten as snugly as is comfortable for the patient, and tie the ends together on the outside just above the stick.

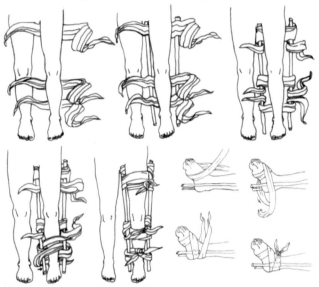

Not only will the stick be immobilized in the wrap; it can rolled up or down to align it vertically. A figure 8 bandage around the foot (lower right) stabilizes the ankle.

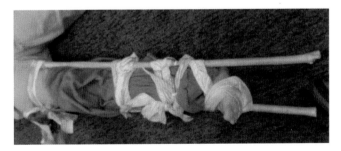

Sticks secured with the swivel hitch can also be swiveled to any angle with the limb - essential if you are splinting a joint injury that locks the limb in a bent position. By securing one or two sticks to the proximal and distal ends of the limb with a swivel hitch, you will complete the third side of the triangle and immobilize the injured joint. Secure the ends of the sticks to the leg near the ankle and the hip with the same technique shown in the previous splint. Lay a wide cravat across the sticks, secure it as shown in the following drawing, and fill the space between the cravat and the back of the knee with padding.

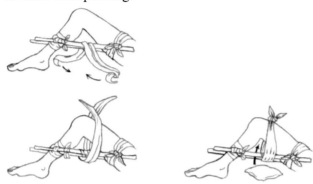

If the patient is on a stretcher or litter, another way to stabilize a locked knee is to lay a rolled blanket or bulky jacket over the good knee, pick up the injured leg (maintaining the angle of the knee) and cross the ankle over the ankle of the uninjured leg, so that the injured knee is supported by the rolled blanket. Then lash the ankles together with a cravat. This splint will stabilize an injured knee while the patient is being evacuated on the stretcher or improvised litter.

An ice ax also makes a good lower leg splint. Put padding (if available) between the shaft and the leg. Immobilize the ankle with a figure 8 bandage - One loop of the figure 8 secures the toe of the boot to the pick of the ax; the other loop wraps the splinted ankle.

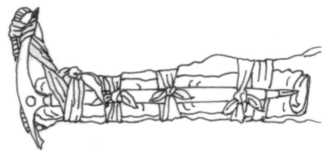

Fractured clavicle

If a clavicle (collarbone) is fractured, a figure 8 bandage that holds the shoulders back in the military at attention position will help stabilize it. Wrap a cravat or piece of webbing around the injured shoulder, cross it in an X on the back, then wrap it around the other shoulder and tie it. A pack with the shoulder straps cinched tight can also serve as a figure 8 bandage. Use

padding under the bandage if it presses uncomfortably on the injured side. While a sling is more comfortable, and preferred by most orthopedists for stabilizing the clavicle as it gradually heals, the figure 8 bandage enables the patient to use both hands while hiking, bicycling, or skiing out of the wilderness.

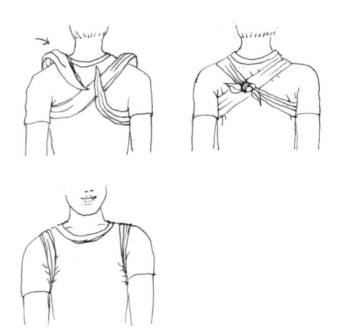

Arm splints

To splint a fractured forearm, you can use a padded stick or pole on the palm side, so that the relaxed fingers either curl around the end or are supported by padding between the palm and the stick. With either technique, you need to immobilize the wrist by wrapping the hand up to the first knuckles. A padded stick or pole can also be used to splint a fractured humerus, by placing it on the outside of the upper arm, where it will be close to the bone.

A padded wire mesh splint or a SAM splint can immobilize an arm fracture more comfortably and securely. First bend it into a half cylinder, then use the uninjured arm to mold it into shape, so that it fits when you apply it to the injured forearm or upper arm

For a forearm or wrist fracture, the sugar tong is he most secure. Measure it on the uninjured arm (flexed at least 90° with the palm parallel to the chest) by wrapping it around the elbow so the splint encloses the forearm on two sides. If there is enough extra on the palm side, roll it up under the palm to hold the hand in the relaxed position of function. If the other side of the splint is long enough, it can go past the wrist to immobilize that joint; or the wrist can be immobilized by wrapping the hand up to the first knuckles.

If the sugar tong presses uncomfortably on the fracture, you can fold the wire mesh or SAM splint double, and place it on the palm side only of the forearm. For either design, you can secure the splint with cravats, bandanas, coban (a self-adhering bandage), or gauze roller bandage. The advantage of gauze rollers is that they are stretchy, so you can wrap the whole splinted forearm without causing discomfort. Do NOT, however, use tape to secure a SAM splint, because when you remove it, the tape will shred the foam padding of the splint.

To splint a fractured humerus with a padded wire mesh or SAM splint, one technique is to fold about a foot of the splint double, then wrap the doubled part around the elbow of the uninjured arm so that it extends part way to the armpit on the inside of the arm. Then fold the single thickness of the splint into a half cylinder and mold it to the outside of the uninjured upper arm, and apply it to the injured upper arm.

After checking distal circulation, sensation, movement and strength (and comparing them to the uninjured arm), you should do three additional tests that check the function of three nerves: ulnar, median, and radial. Ulnar: make a fan with the fingers; median: touch the tip of the thumb to the base of the little finger; radial: extend the fingers and hand. If the patient already is showing wrist drop (cannot extend the wrist at all) then radial nerve function is impaired. Since the radial nerve wraps around the humerus before continuing down the arm, it is most likely to be injured in a humerus fracture. By the time the patient gets to the hospital, distal nerve functions may be impaired by swelling. But if you documented that these functions were unimpaired before and after splinting, then the patient will probably not need surgery to repair the nerves.

Slings

An injured arm, even after being splinted, needs to be supported by a sling, which you can improvise by pulling the bottom of patient's shirt or jacket up around the arm and safety pinning it to itself. A triangular bandage, however, makes a much more versatile sling. Twist the point of the bandage into a rat's tail and tie

an overhand knot in it (or use a safety pin) to create a cup for the elbow. Then ease the triangular bandage between the splinted arm and the patient's chest so that the upper tail goes over the good shoulder, with the knot toward the elbow of the injured arm. Bring up the lower tail to wrap and support the forearm. You have three choices of where to go with that tail before tying it to the other tail:

*   Bring it around the other side of the neck (American style).
*   Bring it around the outside of the injured arm (French style) so it cradles the arm.
*   Bring it under and through the armpit of the injured arm (British style).

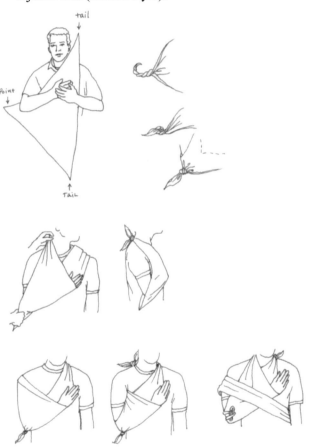

Both the French and British style slings take pressure off the neck and make it easier to get good wrist elevation, which is important for reducing swelling before the arm is put in a cast. Generally, the French style is best for a lower arm fracture. The British style is useful for an upper arm fracture, because it does not put any pressure on the injury.

After tying the sling, secure the arm to the body with a swathe – a cravat bandage or cloth strip wrapped around the arm and the chest to prevent the injured arm from flapping as the patient walks or is transported.

Hand and finger splints

A broken finger can be splinted to one or two adjacent fingers, using athletic tape or a narrow gauze roller to secure it. If possible, keep the finger in the relaxed and slightly flexed position of function. If several fingers or hand bones are broken, you can stabilize the whole hand in the position of function, with the tip of the thumb near the tip of the forefinger, by filling the hollow of the palm with padding or rolled up bandages, then wrapping the whole hand with a stretchy gauze roller or surgical wrap. Anchor the bandage at the wrist, then wrap diagonally over the back and palm sides of the hand to the wrist, gently holding the fingers curled around the padding in the palm. Then wrap diagonally around the palm side and back of the hand to the wrist to secure the remaining fingers, and tie or tape the bandage at the wrist. A sling will support the stabilized hand in comfort.

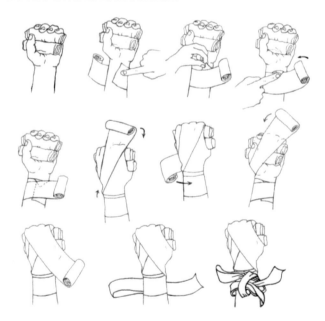

Sprains

In a wilderness activity where participants need the full use of their bodies, ligament tears (sprains) or muscle tears (strains) can be disabling. At best, they will interrupt the trip. At worst, they can turn the trip into a survival situation. By knowing how to assess sprains, you can make an informed decision about what to do.

Can the patient safely continue after a rest or at a reduced level of activity? Is an evacuation necessary? Will the patient need medical treatment to avoid possible loss of function? If the patient has to walk on an injured joint to get out of a hazardous situation, then you need to know how to support and stabilize the joint (e.g., by taping it).

Assessment of ligament damage is easiest shortly after the injury occurs. As the joint begins to swell, it becomes much more difficult to assess function and integrity. If you reduce the swelling in an injured joint, that will help ease the pain, prevent secondary damage, and speed healing. You should also know how to prevent and rehabilitate athletic injuries in yourself.

Swelling impairs circulation and causes pain in an injured joint by compressing blood vessels and nerves. The first goal in treating a sprain, therefore, is to reduce the swelling. The traditional mnemonic is **RICE**: Rest, Ice, Compression, Elevation. Elevating the joint helps drainage, along with compression, and avoids pumping too much blood to an area where it may accumulate and seep into tissues from damaged vessels. Cooling the joint constricts blood vessels and slows the release of synovial fluid.

If ice is available, crush it and seal it in a plastic bag. Apply the ice for 20 minutes every hour. In between the ice packs, apply compression with a wide elastic bandage. If no ice is available, wet the bandage and loosen it between periods of compression. To secure the ice pack, first wrap the elastic bandage loosely around the joint until it is covered. Then apply the ice pack, and continue wrapping the bandage around it until it is secure.

Compression works on a sprain only if it is applied to the swelling. Simply wrapping the joint with an elastic bandage would put most of the pressure on the bony knobs. So cut a horseshoe from a cotton or felt pad at least 1" thick to fit around the kneecap or ankle knob. Fit the horseshoe around the knob so that the open side is towards the heart.

Then wrap the joint with an elastic bandage. When applying compression, check distal circulation and sensation at regular intervals. Test capillary refill in the toenails (or the skin if the patient is wearing nail polish), and compare nerve function. If distal functions are impaired, loosen the bandage.

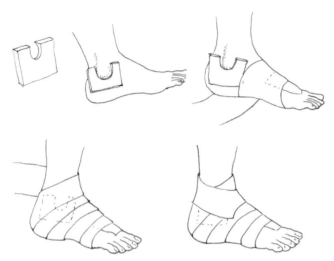

Applying compression between ice to reduce swelling

Rehabilitating sprains

If a sprain is not so severe that it requires surgery, you should begin rehabilitation as soon as the swelling goes down. Immobilized muscles lose strength twice as fast as they regain it after an injury, which delays recovery of full function and increases the chance of re-injury. Physical therapists have a saying about sprains: for every day in the cast, two more days of rehabilitation.

Rehabilitation begins with range of motion exercises. For a sprained ankle, sitting with the leg dangling and writing alphabets with the big toe simulates the joint's natural movements. This exercise can be combined with contrast baths: immersing the ankle alternately in basins of warm and ice-cold water, for a few minutes at a time, as you exercise.

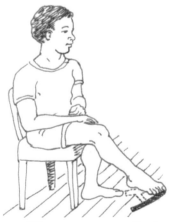

When you can easily do range of motion exercises, begin resistance exercises, using a strip of surgical rubber or a bicycle inner tube. For the ankle, pull the toes up, down and to either side.

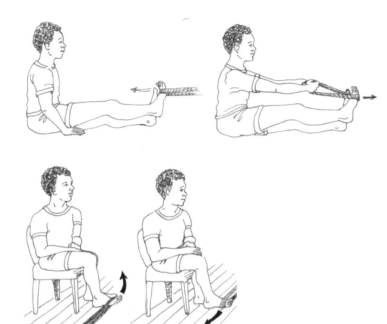

Tubing also works for knee and shoulder exercises, though exercise machines in a gym are more convenient. It is important, however, to keep weight off a sprained ankle or knee until they can bear weight painlessly. Days on crutches can save weeks or months of limping.

Balance exercises are the last stage of rehabilitating a knee or ankle injury. If you can stand on one foot for 30 seconds, you are ready to begin.

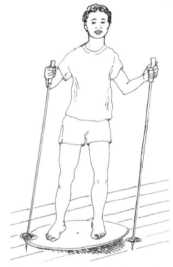

You can make a balance board by cutting an 18" circle from ¾" plywood, then screwing one-half of a wooden ball to the center. Plant your feet on either side of the center and try to balance the board on the ball. If you feel unstable, you can hold a pair of hiking or ski poles for safety, planting them when you are in danger of losing your balance.

Athletes with unstable ankles often tape them before competition. Athletic tape is porous, so that it does not trap moisture on the skin. Taping is designed to limit motions that would pull on loose and weakened ligaments. Usually these are the ligaments on the lateral side of the ankle. Apply vertical and horizontal strips of tape alternately, so that they interlock. Begin with vertical strips on the inside (medial side) of the leg and pull them strongly before sticking them to the outside (lateral side). This will evert the ankle as much as possible. Finish the taping with some diagonal strips. If the tape does not stick well, try wiping tincture of benzoin on the skin first.

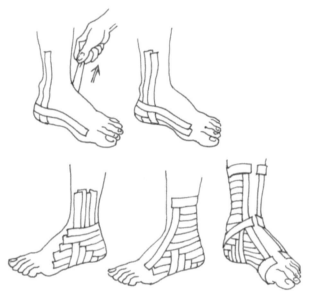

The tape must not circle the ankle or leg completely. Otherwise, it would inhibit circulation as the ankle swells. A strip of bare skin should be on the front of the shin and the top of the foot. This technique is called the Gibney wrap.

Reducing dislocations

If a **finger joint** has been dislocated, at least one ligament is probably completely torn. The finger will be crooked and have a bump at the joint. To put the finger back in joint, flex the finger slightly to relax the tendons; and pull as though you were cracking your knuckles (or the knuckles of your patient.) If the finger is slippery from sweat, wrap it in cloth for traction. Gently press the finger back into joint with your thumb as you pull. After putting the finger back in joint, splint it to prevent re-injury, ideally in the relaxed, slightly flexed, position.

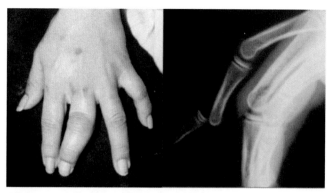

Dislocated finger and x-ray.
Photos courtesy of Ben Schifrin, MD

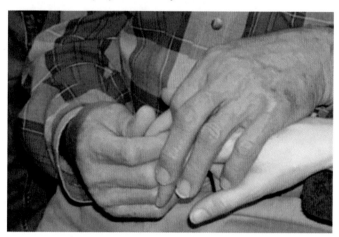

Dr. Serra shows how to reduce a dislocated finger
Photo courtesy of Mark Stinson, MD

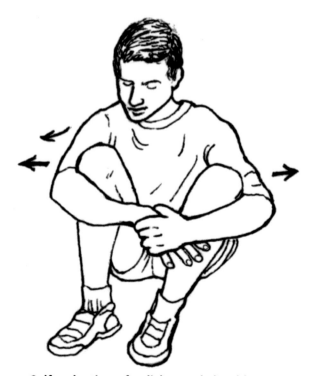

Self-reduction of a dislocated shoulder

When a **shoulder** is dislocated, the knob of the humerus usually pops out in the front of the socket (anterior dislocation), so you can see and feel a lump there, and the arm will be locked in place. The arm will often be held up or away from the body in an awkward position. If the humerus is pulled far enough out to clear the rim of the socket, however, it may slip back in place. A patient who is alone can try **self-reduction.** Wrap the arms around both knees, grip the wrist of the injured arm with the other hand, and spread the legs. This is most likely to work for someone who has suffered chronic shoulder dislocations, because the damage makes the shoulder joint easier both to dislocate and to relocate.

If that doesn't work, and there is a ledge or large fallen tree trunk available, try lying face down on it with the injured arm dangling and a 15-20 pound weight hanging from the arm. You can strap or tape a day pack to the wrist or elbow and fill it with water bottles or rocks. After 20 minutes or so, the muscles should fatigue enough to pull the knob of the humerus past the rim of the joint and let it slip back in.

Another way to reduce a shoulder dislocation is to have the patient lie face up with the injured arm outstretched. Sit down where you can grasp the wrist or arm with both hands, plant the ball of your foot (with the shoe off) in the armpit, then apply traction by leaning back.

If the **kneecap** (Latin *patella:* "a small dish or pan") slides out of position, usually to the outside, it can lock the knee joint. To put it back in place, hold the leg up with one hand under the knee and the other hand gripping the leg near the ankle. Slowly straighten the leg while pushing the kneecap back in place with your thumb.

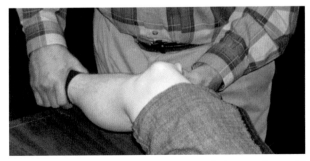

Dr. Serra shows how to reduce a dislocated patella
Photo courtesy of Mark Stinson, MD

If the ankle is dislocated, it will be deformed, and the patient will not be able to move it much. To reduce the dislocation, flex the patient's knee 90° to relax the tendons. Grip the ball of the foot with one hand and lift the foot; let the weight of the leg shift the bones back into place, using the other hand to guide them.

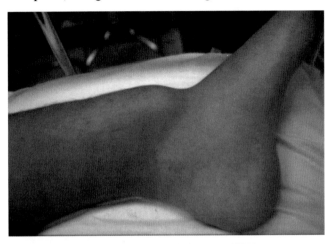

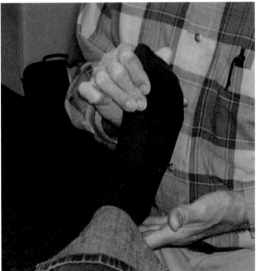

Dr. Serra shows how to reduce an ankle dislocation
Photo courtesy of Mark Stinson, MD

Conclusion

In an urban situation, splints usually have to stay in place only during a short ambulance ride. In the wilderness, however, they usually need to stay on for a long time to protect the injured limb as the patient walks out or is evacuated. So wilderness rescuers need to know how to construct good splints with whatever materials they carry or can improvise on the scene. They also need to know how to assess, treat, and rehabilitate sprains and common dislocations.

Chapter 7. Injuries affecting vital organs and functions

Head injuries

Under the scalp is a network of blood vessels which can bleed copiously from a wound. But any blood accumulating inside the skull will compress the brain. As intracranial pressure (ICP) increases, the patient's level of responsiveness will decline, and other vital functions (breathing, pulse, and blood pressure) may change.

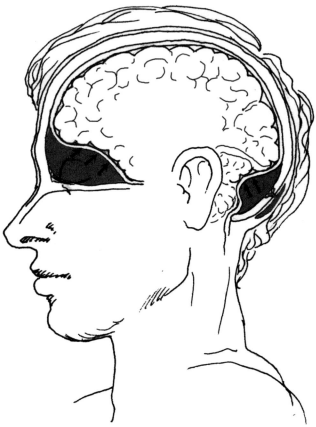

In a wilderness accident, you need to assess patients for head injuries, recognize the signs of skull fracture or concussion, and record the symptoms of brain injury.

Scalp wounds

If there are no signs of a skull fracture, use direct pressure on the wound to control bleeding. If there are signs of a skull fracture, pull the wound edges together by grasping tufts of long hair on either side, then tie the tufts together over a dressing. For someone with short or no hair, you can pull the edges of the wound together with tape. If bleeding is not severe and there is no sign of a skull fracture, clean the wound by irrigating it and protect it with a sterile dressing, just as with any other wound.

Skull fracture

When you examine the head (see the patient assessment chapter) look for any open wound, blood, or deformity. Then feel the skull, gently, for any deformity. Check the eyes and behind the ears. If an artery between the dura mater and the skull is ruptured by a skull fracture, blood can seep into the tissues around the eyes (raccoon eyes) or behind the ears (Battle's sign), giving them a bruised appearance. Raccoon eyes are a more common sign of skull fracture than bruising behind the ears, and can appear soon after the accident if bleeding inside the skull is severe.

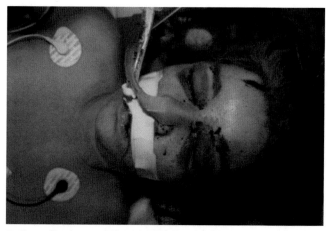

Fallen climber with a skull fracture & raccoon eyes
Photo courtesy of Ben Schifrin, MD

Cerebrospinal fluid (CSF), which bathes and cushions the brain and spinal cord, may leak out of the ears or nose. It is a clear fluid, like raw egg white. If blood is coming out of the nose or ears, capture some on a gauze pad or piece of cloth. Blood alone will spread into a uniform, dark red patch. CSF in the blood will form a yellow ring around the patch. Leaking CSF means that the patient has a skull fracture.

Assessing brain functions

Always ask anyone who has had a fall or collision:
- Did you hit your head?
- Did you lose consciousness?

- Do you have any pain in your head or neck?

If the patient is not sure, try to reconstruct the sequence of events. Any gap in the story suggests temporarily altered consciousness, amnesia, or both. After checking the skull for blood and deformity, check the eyes for:
- Pupil size (Unequal? Both dilated?)
- Light response (Slow? Absent?)
- Vision ("How many fingers?")
- Motion ("Without moving your head, follow my fingers with your eyes.")

Some people have naturally unequal pupils, but if one pupil is completely dilated, then there is an injury on that side of the brain putting pressure on the cranial nerve. Dilation is the relaxed position of the iris muscle, and the motor nerves to the eye, including the pupil, are the only ones that do not cross. You may also find loss of function on the opposite side of the face and body, as with a stroke. Does the patient feel any tingling or numbness? Check and compare sensation ("Which finger am I touching?"), movement, and strength on both sides of the body. Record the results and note the time. Also keep checking responsiveness by talking to the patient and record the results regularly. The only way to save a patient who is becoming less responsive because of bleeding inside the skull is by rapid evacuation to a hospital where brain surgery can relieve the pressure.

Concussion

Even if the skull is not fractured, a blow to the head can bounce the brain inside and rupture blood vessels. This injury is called a concussion (Latin *concussus* "shaken violently"). Effects of a concussion may include loss of consciousness, amnesia, and blurred or double vision as well as dizziness, balance problems, and nausea. Any blow to the head that causes changes in brain functions is serious, and if brain functions are deteriorating, then the patient's condition is critical. It is especially dangerous for someone who has had one blow to the head to risk another impact.

A concussion that causes a slow bleed inside the skull can have delayed effects, days or weeks later. Headache is the most common symptom (50% of cases). Other symptoms may include neck pain, ringing in the ears, dizziness, or drowsiness. Behavioral effects may include depression, loss of emotional control, anxiety, irritability, sleep disturbances and

hypersensitivity to noise or light. The patient may also have cognitive problems including loss of memory, concentration or attention.

Recent studies of concussions in contact sports like football have used brain scans to reveal neurological damage. Researchers thought that the scans would show a difference between players who had been diagnosed with concussions, and those who had not. But the scans showed damage in the brains of all the players. So impacts to the head can have lasting effects even if there have been no obvious signs of concussion or intracranial bleeding.

What can you do?

Recognizing head injuries and assessing the damage are important skills for wilderness first aiders, because they enable you to make prompt decisions about evacuation. You also need to watch and guard the patient's airway, because head injury patients may vomit. Be ready to clear out the vomitus before it can be sucked into the lungs, using a suction device or cloth. After taking spinal precautions, put the patient in a head-up position if possible, with the body elevated about 30° to help relieve pressure inside the skull.

Eye injuries

The most common eye problem is a foreign body on the surface. Even a small speck on the surface will be irritating. If blinking doesn't remove the irritant, try irrigating the eye with sterile saline, or disinfected water. Squirt from the inside corner with the head tilted to let fluid drain downward. Another technique is to grasp the lashes of the upper lid and pull it outward and down over the lower lid. If the speck sticks to the inside of the upper lid, it may then adhere to the outside of the lower lid.

If a foreign body will not come off the eye's surface or is embedded, protect the eye and evacuate the patient. An eye patch should cover the eye without touching it. The patch should have a pinhole in the center, which will admit light and help to keep the eye focused straight ahead. Also use eye patches for penetrating eye injuries or a blow to the eye that causes bleeding in the anterior chamber. If the lid is injured, so that it cannot spread tears over the surface, keep the eye moist with sterile saline or disinfected water.

Eye infections

Eye irritation may be caused by allergies that are known to the patient. But an eye infection requires medical care. Signs and symptoms may include a pink or red appearance of the white of the eye caused by inflammation, itching, tearing, pus, crusted eyelashes, or lids stuck together in the morning. Rinsing the eye several times a day with sterile saline or disinfected water may help.

Contact lenses

Any injury or medical problem that interferes with circulation or dehydrates the patient can dry out the eye and cause the contact lens to adhere. So you may have to remove the lenses as a precaution, especially in an unresponsive patient. A contact lens container and a small sealed bottle of sterile saline in your first aid kit will enable you to store and safeguard the lenses, though the patient may have these. To remove hard or soft lenses, use a mini-marshmallow. Pull it in half to create a sticky surface, and use it to capture and slide out the lens. The sugar in the marshmallow will not harm the lens or the eye.

Nosebleeds

Minor bleeding from the nose can often be controlled by pinching the narrow part of the nose, which puts pressure on the small arteries. Keep up the pressure for 10-15 minutes. A spring-loaded clothes pin or binder clip (with padding underneath) can replace finger pressure. For more serious bleeding, have the patient sit leaning forward and spitting out blood to prevent blood from trickling into the air passages or making the patient nauseated. But a patient with a nosebleed that will not stop should be evacuated.

Dental injuries

Any trauma that damages teeth can also damage the head or face. Check for **associated injuries** which may be more dangerous, no matter how distracting the dental pain is. Did the patient lose consciousness during or after the accident? Are vision and eye movement normal?

If the lower jaw is fractured, you may feel a step deformity in the bone, or notice the teeth on that side are misaligned. If the jaw hinge fractures, it will be difficult and painful for the patient to move the jaw. Stabilize a fractured jaw with a jaw bandage. Tie a half-bow for quick release, in case the patient becomes nauseated.

Broken teeth

If only the tooth's outside layer of hard white enamel is broken, the damage is minor. If the yellow dentin under the enamel is broken, the patient may feel considerable pain. If the red pulp is damaged, the patient will feel intense pain, and the tooth may become infected. Any fractured tooth that exposes the pulp requires rapid evacuation and dental surgery. Exposed dentin as well as pulp is very sensitive. Air and temperature change can both cause pain.

Temporary filling

If the patient loses a filling or cracks the tooth without exposing the pulp, a temporary filling (such as Cavit dental filling paste or sugar-free gum) will protect it and possibly reduce the pain. It will also round off any jagged edges left by the break, preventing lacerations of the tongue and mouth. If you are not sure which tooth is hurting, you can locate the pain by tapping on teeth in the affected area.

Knocked out teeth

If an adult tooth is knocked out, you can try to re-implant it. A tooth properly re-implanted within 30 minutes has a 50% chance of survival. After two hours out of the socket, however, its chances drop below 10%. Hold the tooth only by the crown (the part that is normally visible when the tooth is in its socket). Use sterile gloves, if you have them. Do not touch the root. If the tooth is dirty, rinse it with sterile saline solution (not plain water). If you don't have saline, use milk or the patient's saliva. Never scrub the tooth, however, because it would damage cells on the root's surface.

Spinal injuries

The seven cervical vertebrae are the most vulnerable to injury because the neck gives them little support or protection. Any vertebra can be injured by a direct blow, but cervical vertebrae can be injured by a blow to the top of the head as well. Cervical vertebrae are also vulnerable to bending and twisting forces, which can tear the ligaments that hold the vertebrae together. If enough of these ligaments are torn, the vertebrae become unstable. If a vertebra shifts sideways by one-third of its diameter, it will sever the spinal cord.

The twelve thoracic vertebrae are attached to the ribs, so that the rib cage helps to stabilize them. The lumbar spine in the lower back, with five vertebrae, is stabilized by the strong muscles of the abdomen and lower back. It can be injured by a radiating force from a hard fall on the tail bone as well as by a direct blow. The five sacral vertebrae are fused together in the pelvis.

The spinal cord is a continuation of the lower brain (the medulla oblongata). It is bathed in and cushioned by the same cerebrospinal fluid as the brain and sealed in protective membranes (dura), which are contiguous with the membranes around the brain. Nerve roots branch out from the spinal cord to either side, between each pair of vertebrae. Sensory and motor nerves proliferate from the nerve roots.

If the spinal cord is pinched, bruised, or cut by an injury, its functions will be impaired below that point. The patient may feel tingling and numbness or have complete loss of sensation. Loss of motor function may range from weakness to complete paralysis. Even if the patient is paralyzed, however, the damage may not be permanent. If the spinal cord is bruised or pinched rather than cut, the patient may recover, provided that rescuers protect the spine from further injury.

Spinal assessment

As with any possible injury, try to reconstruct and visualize the mechanism – could it have caused a spinal injury? Patient assessment includes head-to-toe exam, vital signs, and medical history. When doing the head-to-toe exam, you may be able to feel deformity in vertebrae with your fingertips or elicit point tenderness with gentle pressure, as with any bone injury. Ask if there is any pain or discomfort in the neck or the rest of the spine, and if so can the patient tell you where it hurts. Also, the patient may have a stiff neck. The absence of these signs and symptoms, however, does not rule out a spinal injury, especially if there are signs or symptoms of serious head or face injury.

If you suspect spinal injury, it is especially important to check neurological function in the fingers and toes: sensation, movement and strength. To test

sensation, ask: "Which finger (or toe) am I touching?" and block the patient's view to make sure that you get an honest response. Try a soft touch first, with your fingertip. If that gets no response, try a sharp touch with your fingernail or a pin. Then, if there are no bone or joint injuries in the limb, ask the patient to wiggle the fingers (or toes). To test and compare strength in the hands, have the patient grip your two crossed fingers with each hand and squeeze. With each foot, have the patient push down, then up, against your hand. Always test and compare both sides.

Loss of function on one side of the body may be from a brain injury or stroke. Spinal injuries affect both sides of the body equally. In cold weather, however, hypothermia or frostbite may be interfering with neurological functions and masking the effects of a possible spinal injury.

Although a spinal injury may cause loss of voluntary movement to some parts of the body, they may still move reflexively in response to a stimulus. Normally the nervous signal would pass through the brain, which would moderate the response. If the reflex is exaggerated, and uncontrolled, this suggests spinal injury. For example, a tap below the kneecap may cause the leg to jerk up violently. Or the patient may show priapism (uncontrolled erection).

Clearing the spine

In a wilderness accident, you are unlikely to have the equipment to immobilize the spine during evacuation. You also may not be in a place where you can bivouac and wait for rescue. So it is important to be able to rule out spinal injury (clear the spine), if possible, in a wilderness accident. Even for urban situations, some emergency medical systems in the U.S. are now training EMTs to clear the spine. The mnemonic for the kind of patient you need to clear the spine is PASS.

- A reasonably **pain-free** patient. Any painful injury, such as a fracture, deep laceration, or serious burn, may mask the pain of a spinal injury.
- An **alert** and fully responsive patient who can give reliable answers to your questions. If the patient is not fully responsive because of a head injury, heat illness, hypothermia, altitude illness, or a medical problem, then you cannot clear the spine.
- A **sober** patient. Alcohol, recreational drugs and some medications can alter mental functions or

suppress pain. If the patient is experiencing such effects, you cannot clear the spine.

- A **sane** patient. Patients who are mentally disturbed may not give reliable answers.

Once the patient passes the pre-test, you can verify good spinal functions: sensation, movement, and strength. If the patient has any tingling or numbness, any loss of sensation, movement, or strength that is on both sides, then you cannot clear the spine. If the patient has any neck pain or stiffness, you cannot clear the cervical spine. Similarly, if the patient has any pain or stiffness in the lower body (not accounted for by local injuries), you cannot clear the spine. But if you have done a thorough spinal assessment, and found no signs or symptoms of spinal injury, you can do final tests to clear the spine. Caution the patient to stop if it hurts, and:

- Turn the head from side to side (rotate).
- Put the chin on one shoulder, then the other.
- Lift the chin and look up (extend).
- Put the chin down on the chest (flex).

If the patient can do all of these movements without pain, stiffness, or discomfort, then in a wilderness situation, you can clear the spine. To rule out a possible injury to the lumbar spine, have the patient twist from side to side, stretch sideways in both directions, bend backwards, and then bend forwards from the waist – again cautioning the patient to stop if it hurts.

Chest injuries

Most chest and abdominal injuries in wilderness activities are caused by impact from falls or collisions. Reconstruct the mechanism of injury and ask yourself what damage it could have caused. For example, a rock climber who did a long pendulum and smashed against the rock sideways may have cracked ribs or fractured the pelvis, and the impact (or the broken bone ends) may have ruptured blood vessels or vital organs.

Monitor the effects of the accident on the patient's vital systems, especially if they suggest shock. Vital signs may change because of direct damage to the vital organ in question. For example, breathing may change, because a lung has been torn open by a cracked rib. They may also change from the indirect effects of damage elsewhere. For example, internal loss of blood,

which reduces circulation, can change skin signs and level of responsiveness as well as pulse and breathing.

Signs and symptoms in a patient with a chest injury that impairs breathing may include:

- guarding or self-splinting position;
- asymmetrical chest movement;
- rapid breathing;
- labored breathing with use of accessory muscles (tensed neck muscles, flared nostrils);
- voluntary restriction of breathing;
- air under the skin (crackly to the touch);
- cyanosis (blue lips, gums, skin);
- coughing up blood;
- distended veins in neck;
- rapid pulse (especially over 130 per minute).

Chest injuries can interfere with breathing and circulation by impairing chest movement, collapsing a lung, bruising the heart, or compressing the heart inside its protective sack with accumulating blood.

If you visualize the mechanism of breathing, then the possible effects of a chest injury on respiration will be easier to assess. The lungs are enclosed in a slippery membrane that is normally pressed against a membrane lining the inside of the chest cavity by air pressure inside the lung. This air pressure varies as you inhale and exhale, but as long as no air or blood gets between lungs and chest wall, the lungs should remain inflated.

When the rib cage expands and the diaphragm flattens, the lungs expand with the chest cavity. Since the volume of the lungs has increased, air pressure inside drops below atmospheric pressure, and new air flows in through the airways. When the chest contracts and the relaxed diaphragm domes up, they compress the air inside the lungs and force some of it out. The lungs also contract because of their elasticity.

What can interfere with this mechanism for moving air in and out of the lungs? If a lung is punctured by a cracked rib, then the lung will begin to collapse like a balloon with a slow leak. This is called a **pneumothorax** (Greek *pneuma* "air" *thorax* "chest"). Blood leaking between the lung and the chest wall can have a similar effect, called **hemothorax** ("blood in the chest"). If the chest wall is pierced, and the hole is too big to be self-sealing, then air will be sucked in through the hole when you expand the chest, collapsing the lung. This is called a **sucking chest wound**. Another injury that will impair breathing is an impact that fractures many ribs and breaks loose a whole section of the rib cage – at least three ribs broken in at least two places (**flail chest**). When the chest contracts, the broken section will be pushed out by the increasing air pressure inside the lungs, and it will be pushed in when the chest expands (**paradoxical motion**). By reducing the effective volume of the expanded chest cavity, this injury reduces the amount of air moved in and out with each breath. It is called flail chest because of the flail-like motion of the broken section. Similarly, an injury to the heart that causes bleeding inside its protective sack will gradually compress the heart and reduce the amount of blood that it can receive from the veins and pump out

When assessing a patient with a possible chest injury, always go to skin and check for bruising, crackling or an open wound. Rule out spinal injury if you can, because spinal precautions would limit your options and make rescue much more difficult. Also, backboarding would restrict breathing already compromised by the chest injury.

Usually a patient with breathing problems will be more comfortable, and able to breathe better, in a sitting position. But a patient with an injury to one side of the chest who cannot or does not want to sit up should be placed on the injured side to protect the good lung. You should give oxygen (if you have it) to any patient in respiratory distress, and protect the airway.

Children and chest injuries

Since children's bones have less mineral content than adult bones, they are more flexible. As a result, their rib cages flex more with the impact of a fall or collision, and transmit more of the impact to internal organs. So even if a child seems all right after blunt chest trauma, it is important to watch vital signs over the next day or two, because a slow air leak or bleed may happen inside the chest. If the child's vital signs do start to change (e.g., more rapid breathing and pulse), then you should assume that a chest injury has occurred and evacuate.

Rib fractures and separations

Any fall or collision with an impact to the rib cage can damage it. A cracked rib, like any fracture, usually causes a sharp, local pain, and point tenderness when touched. Moving, straining, twisting, or coughing can cause severe pain. You can locate rib fractures during patient assessment by putting gentle hand pressure on the sides of the rib cage, then asking the patient to take a deep breath and point to where it hurts.

An impact on the rib cage can tear the cartilage that connects the ribs (separation). An extensive tear is very painful and slow to heal. It can cause severe pain whenever the patient makes a move that pulls on the torn cartilage, e.g., lying down or getting up, coughing, or sometimes just taking a deep breath.

Emergency care for either injury is to keep the patient comfortable, check for effects on breathing and circulation, and try to prevent further damage, especially to the lungs. It is usually not helpful to tape or splint the ribs. In fact, it may be harmful by restricting breathing even more than the patient will be doing voluntarily.

Pneumothorax and hemothorax

Young people, especially tall thin men who smoke, as well as people with emphysema can get blebs (blisters) or cysts on the lungs that can cause air leaks when they rupture (**spontaneous pneumothorax**). An impact to the chest, or the jagged ends of broken ribs, can also cause an air leak by tearing the lung. Usually the patient will feel a sharp pain in the chest that gets worse with inhaling. As the lung shrinks, the patient will feel short of breath and breathe faster. A patient who cannot sit up should be placed on the injured side to protect the lung that is still functioning.

If the tear acts like a one-way flap valve, then the increasing air pressure in the injured side of the chest will collapse the lung: **tension pneumothorax**. The trachea may eventually be twisted to the side by the unequal pressure; and pressure on the heart reduces the return of blood to the heart, so the jugular veins in the neck will become distended. Bleeding into the chest cavity (hemothorax) has similar effects. In both cases, you need to evacuate as rapidly as possible and give oxygen if you have it.

Sucking chest wound

If an open wound penetrates the chest and is too wide to self-seal, you will see air bubbling through the blood, and you may hear a sucking sound as the patient inhales. You need to seal the hole immediately with a gloved hand as another rescuer prepares an air-proof patch. If you are alone, have the patient hold a hand over the wound if possible while you prepare the patch.

Your patch should be at least three or four times as big as the hole - otherwise it might be sucked in. A plastic baggie, secured with duct tape over a layer of sterile gauze makes a good air-proof patch. If possible, leave one side of the patch untaped so that it will act as a one-way flutter valve.

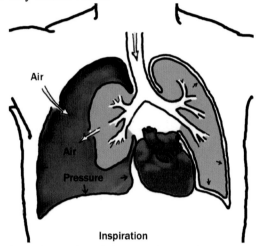

Inspiration

When the patient inhales, the patch will be pulled in and sealed by the difference in air pressure. When the patient exhales, some air may be forced out on the untapped side, slightly reducing the pressure inside the chest.

Flail chest

If multiple fractures have broken loose a segment of the rib cage, the muscles may self-splint the injury until they tire. Then you will see the paradoxical motion of a flail chest - a section bulging out when the patient exhales, and pulled inward as the patient inhales and expands the chest. You will also see signs and symptoms of respiratory distress. While the patient may feel more comfortable holding or lying on a cushion over the injury, trying to splint it will probably do more harm than good by further restricting breathing that is already impaired. Aside from oxygen, the only treatment is rapid evacuation.

Cardiac tamponade

Since the heart is enclosed in a tough sack called the pericardium (Greek *peri* "around" *kardia* "heart"), bleeding inside the sack will compress the heart and reduce the amount of blood it can take in and pump out. Cardiac tamponade (French *tampon* "to plug up") is usually caused by a penetrating wound that seals up,.

But it can also be caused by a hard impact to the chest that bruises the heart.

The pulse will become rapid and weak as the heart speeds up to compensate for reduced stroke volume. Pulse pressure (the difference between systolic and diastolic pressure) will narrow as systolic pressure decreases. Heart sounds will become muffled. Jugular veins will become distended from back pressure in blood returning to the compressed heart. You should give the patient oxygen if you have it and evacuate as rapidly as possible.

Abdominal injuries

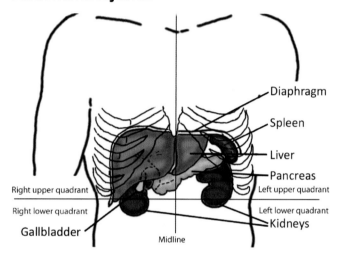

Falls and impacts as well as penetrating wounds can injure abdominal organs. **Solid, blood-filled organs**, especially the liver and spleen, can bleed enough when they are ruptured to send the patient quickly into shock. A blow to the upper abdomen, just below the rib notch, or a blow that fractures ribs on the lower right side of the chest, can rupture the liver. About 20% of patients with multiple rib fractures on the lower left side of the chest have ruptured spleens. The patient may feel referred pain in the left shoulder (Kerr's sign). If the kidneys are ruptured, the patient will probably feel lower back pain and may have blood in the urine.

Hollow organs, such as the stomach, intestines, and bladder, may be full or empty. The stomach secretes digestive juices which are very irritating to the peritoneum, a membrane that surrounds the abdominal organs(Greek *tonos* "stretching" *peri* "around"); so rupture of the stomach causes severe pain.

Ruptured intestines can release a semi-liquid mixture of food, enzymes, and bacteria that will cause

84

inflammation. Usually the patient will feel a spreading pain and tenderness from the site of the injury. As damaged intestines fill with gas and fluid, the abdomen may distend, and you may feel a guarding reaction - rigid abdominal muscles that the patient cannot relax.

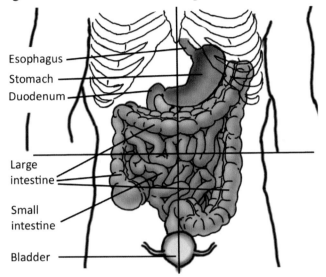

Esophagus
Stomach
Duodenum
Large intestine
Small intestine
Bladder

Blood may appear in the feces. If it is bright red, it is probably from hemorrhoids, but dark tarry blood that is partially digested suggests bleeding in the intestines or stomach.

If the urinary bladder is full, it is more likely to be ruptured by an impact, and it can also be detached from the urethra. This will prevent the patient from urinating. The urinary bladder and the bowel can also be damaged in a pelvis fracture, either directly by the impact or by broken bone ends in the pelvic girdle. If you suspect abdominal injury, always go to skin and check the sides and back as well as the abdomen for any bruising or abrasions.

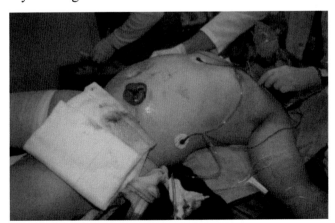

Abdominal injury with protruding intestine.
Photo courtesy of Ben Schifrin, MD

Impaled objects

Immobilize an impaled object with bulky dressings, because trying to pull it out could cause more damage to internal organs as well as more serious bleeding. The only exception would be something going through the cheeks, which you should pull out because it could compromise the airway, and protecting the airway is the highest priority.

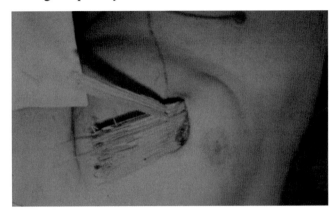

A piece of wood has penetrated the chest wall.
Photo courtesy of Ben Schifrin, MD

Pelvic fracture

An impact to the pelvis from a fall or collision can fracture pelvic bones, which can then lacerate abdominal organs or blood vessels. If the patient shows signs of hypovolemic shock from blood loss, apply a pelvic sling, which goes around the pelvis between the iliac crests and the hip joints. Improvise a pelvic sling from a jacket or sheet. Wrap it around the pelvis (you may have to logroll the patient to get it underneath) and tie the ends together with a sturdy stick or pole in the knot, like an improvised tourniquet. Twist and secure the stick to apply pressure to the pelvis.

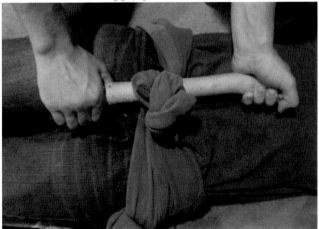

Chapter 8. Medical problems in the wilderness

Respiratory illness

When people get cold, wet, fatigued, or stressed, their resistance is reduced. Also, if one person on a wilderness trip has a respiratory infection, others in the group are liable to pick it up as they share tents and food. So you need to recognize the different types of respiratory illness, distinguish the minor from the more serious that may require evacuation, and know what you can do for the patient.

Respiratory system defenses

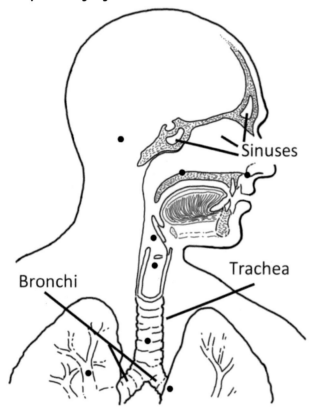

The hairs inside the nostrils are the first line of defense against inhaled dust, which may be contaminated with microorganisms. Then passage into the large sinus (Latin "hollow") behind the nose causes turbulence which tends to carry dust to the sticky mucus membranes. The trachea is also coated with mucus carried slowly upward by the movements of hair-like cilia. There are nerve endings in and behind the nose that trigger a sneeze, and in the airways and lungs that trigger a cough (black dots), when enough mucus accumulates. There are also sneeze triggers in each of the Eustachian tubes between the middle ear and the upper airway. This is a crude reflex for expelling inhaled contaminants. But anything that irritates the walls of the sinuses or air passages, such as cold and dry air, can also trigger mucus production and the sneeze or cough reflex.

Upper respiratory infections

Over-production of mucus in reaction to an infection causes congestion, and swelling of the air passages may further narrow them. This can make it hard to breathe, especially when you lie down to sleep so sleeping in a semi-sitting position may help. The body may react to the infection by raising its temperature (fever). Traditional remedies of staying warm and drinking plenty of fluids may help, and some medications can reduce symptoms such as congestion. Since they can be spread by aerosol as well as by direct or indirect contact, active upper respiratory infections are very contagious.

Middle respiratory infections

So long as a respiratory infection is confined to the upper airways, the patient may feel well enough to continue the trip. Any infection of the bronchi, however, is much more serious. These infections are called bronchitis, and 90% of them are caused by viruses, which antibiotics do not affect. Generally, anyone who is coughing (rather than just sneezing) should not be exercising. Typically, the patient has a deep, racking cough that may be dry (especially at high altitude) or may bring up yellow or greenish mucus. With enough congestion, the patient may be struggling for breath. Anyone in this condition should be evacuated.

Pneumonia

The word "pneumonia" means "disease of the lung," and is a blanket term for any inflammation of the lung. Inflammation is a response of the body that includes diluting fluid, so it can flood the alveoli in which oxygen moves to the blood. The more alveoli are flooded, the less oxygen can move through the lungs. Vomitus aspirated into the lungs can cause pneumonia as well as bacteria and viruses.

Signs and symptoms that distinguish pneumonia from upper respiratory infections may include:

- shaking chills;
- chest pain (sharp rather than dull);
- shortness of breath;
- hot dry skin;
- high temperature.

The patient will probably have a deep, racking cough and should be encouraged to sit up and cough regularly, in order to reduce congestion. An upright position will minimize flooding of the oxygen-exchange surface, because of the shape of the lungs. Anyone with pneumonia should be evacuated because it could be fatal in the wilderness.

Asthma

Asthma (Greek "gasping or panting") attacks can be allergic reactions (about 80%), responses to irritants, or reactions to stress. They can be caused by:

- pollen or other allergens;
- dust;
- pollutants;
- sleeping in a moldy tent;
- food or lotion to which the patient is sensitized;
- cold air;
- exercise.

According to the Center for Disease Control (www.cdc.gov), about 26 million people in the United States suffer from asthma, including over 7 million children, and the percentage of people with asthma is increasing more than exposure to air pollution and other irritants can explain. According to the hygiene hypothesis, an overly clean environment in early childhood prevents the immune system from developing normally, so that it over-reacts when it is later exposed to dust or other irritants. Many athletes have asthma, including Mark Spitz (who won several Olympic gold medals in swimming). So asthma need not prevent people from enjoying outdoor activities if they carry their medications.

In an asthma attack, the respiratory system over-reacts to an irritant, allergen, or stress. Release of chemicals called histamines causes the air passages to constrict, swell, and congest. As in anaphylaxis, the effect can be dramatic. Since airflow is proportional to the fourth power of the passage's radius, reducing the air passage to one-half of its radius (for example) reduces airflow to one-sixteenth. The victim will be in obvious respiratory distress, wheezing and struggling for breath. Asthma kills 5,000 people per year in the United States, and the number is increasing.

As with anaphylactic shock, the only way to relieve a severe asthma attack is with a medication that opens the air passages, reversing the effect of the histamines. These prescription medications, such as albuterol®, are sold as inhalers. Antihistamines, as the name implies, help suppress the production of more histamines, so they supplement asthma inhalers. If you are leading a wilderness trip, medical screening should include questions about asthma and what medications an asthmatic is carrying.

Chronic respiratory diseases

Over 12 million adults in the United States have Chronic Obstructive Pulmonary Disease (**COPD**), and it is the fourth leading cause of death. Smoking is the biggest risk factor, especially for **emphysema** (Greek *emphysan* "to inflate"). In healthy lungs, the elasticity of lung tissue causes it to recoil and expel air when the respiratory muscles are relaxed after breathing in.

Smoking causes chronic narrowing of the airways by inflammation, which makes it harder to exhale – the increased air pressure stretches the elastic walls of the alveoli (**hyperinflation**). In people with advanced emphysema many alveolar walls are destroyed, so that parts of the lungs become dead air spaces, and the lungs are enlarged. They are sometimes described as having barrel chests, because the chest becomes almost as deep as it is wide. They tend to be chronically short of breath, because the large volume of trapped air reduces the amount of fresh air they can inhale.

Patients with COPD may use **accessory muscles** attached to the clavicles and the top of the sternum to help lift the rib cage – you can see these muscles standing out in the neck when they breathe. You may also see **retractions** when they inhale – indentations above the clavicles and between the ribs. They may sit in the **tripod position** – leaning forward with the arms outstretched and the chin forward so as to use the muscles of the abdomen and the back to help them exhale. As they exhale, they may purse their lips to keep up the air pressure and prevent collapse of the bronchial walls. You may also see jugular vein distension (JVD) when the patient exhales, because the increased pressure in the chest from forceful exhaling compresses the heart and reduces venous return, causing back pressure in the veins.

Smoking or air pollution can also cause **chronic bronchitis** by irritating the trachea and bronchi and stimulating the production of excess mucus as well as swelling that narrows the airways. The patient will be coughing frequently to bring up the mucus and clear the airways. Persistent bronchitis can destroy the cilia that line the airways – hair-like cells that carry mucus up to where it can be expelled by coughing.

Tuberculosis

According to the Center for Disease Control (www.cdc.gov), one-third of the world's population is infected with tuberculosis (TB), which is caused by a bacterium: *Mycobacterium tuberculosis*. The bacteria usually attack the lungs (although they can attack other parts of the body as well), so they spread by aerosol when someone with an active infection coughs, sneezes, or speaks. In most of those infected, however, TB is latent, and they are not contagious. But any weakening of the immune system can make someone vulnerable to TB infection or allow a latent infection to become active. HIV infection is a risk factor, but so are diabetes, alcoholism, and smoking.

Worldwide, about 8 million active cases of TB are reported each year (though probably many cases are not reported) and about 10,000 are reported in the United States. TB is still the most deadly infectious disease, killing about 2 million people per year. Although there are now drugs for treating TB, multi-drug resistant strains are becoming more common, as patients may stop taking medications when they feel better, but before the infection is completely cleared. Since patients need to take several drugs daily for 4 to 9 months to be cured (even if TB is still latent), it is not surprising that many do not complete the regimen.

TB was for much of its history called consumption, because it seemed to consume the patient. Signs and symptoms include weight loss and anorexia, fatigue, fever and night sweats as well as coughing and chest pain. Coughing up blood is the classic sign familiar from portrayals of TB in literature and period films. Treatment before effective drugs was a regimen of fresh air and exercise at a sanitarium, supervised by doctors. TB sanitariums, many of them in the mountains, became popular in the second half of the 19th century and did not go completely out of fashion for a century.

Health care workers may be required to have a TB test before working in an ambulance or hospital. The tests are only about 80% sensitive, however, which means they do not detect about 20% of TB infections. Also, the skin test can give a false positive for those who have been vaccinated. Studies on the safety and efficacy of the vaccine show very mixed results, however, so it is not recommended except for people who have serious exposure to TB. Protection from infection includes a HEPA (High Efficiency Particulate Air) respirator.

Heart attack

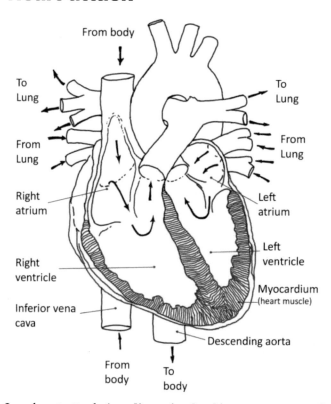

In a heart attack (**cardiogenic shock**), one or more of the arteries supplying the heart muscle with blood is constricted or obstructed. Even if the patient is still breathing and has a pulse, the heart muscle will be damaged, and may be pumping less blood with each contraction. Usually the circulatory system will compensate (as in hypovolemic shock) by withdrawing circulation from the skin (making it cool, pale and clammy) and from the skeletal muscles (which will make the patient feel weak). If the digestive system is deprived of circulation, the patient may become nauseated and vomit, so you need to protect the airway.

The pulse may be weak or irregular. Damage to the left side of the heart can cause back pressure in the pulmonary veins returning oxygenated blood from the lungs to the heart (**congestive heart failure**). Then fluid will accumulate in the lungs (pulmonary edema). Breathing rate may increase to compensate for less oxygen getting through soggy lung tissue to the blood, and you may be able to hear crackles with a stethoscope as small airways open during inhalation and close during exhalation.

The patient may feel a dull pain or discomfort that does not subside. It is usually in the chest, but may radiate down the left arm, or be referred – felt in the jaw or back. Some patients, however, feel no pain from a heart attack, especially if they are elderly. Any exertion could cause a second, probably fatal heart attack. So the most important thing you can do for them is to persuade them not to exert themselves, and wait for evacuation.

Usually a conscious patient suffering a heart attack will be most comfortable in a sitting or semi-sitting position, especially in congestive heart failure, because that position drains the fluid to the bottom of the lungs; whereas lying down would spread the fluid over more lung surface and reduce oxygen delivery to the blood. So give oxygen if you have it. An unresponsive patient who is breathing can be propped in a semi-sitting position.

Stroke

In a stroke, so called because it can be such a sudden affliction, circulation to part of the brain is disrupted by a clot or rupture of a cerebral artery. In an **ischemic stroke** (Greek *ischano*, "I hold in check"), the artery is blocked by a clot. This can happen in two ways:
- An embolus (Greek *embolos* "wedge or plug") forms in the artery.
- A thrombus (Greek *thrombos* "lump or clump") moving from a larger upstream artery jams a smaller branching artery.

In a **hemorrhagic stroke** (Greek *haima* "blood" + *regnumai* "to break forth"), a cerebral artery ruptures. The patient usually gets a sudden and severe headache. With an ischemic stroke caused by a thrombus, the patient may have a headache, because the blockage is sudden; but ischemic strokes from a gradually forming embolus seldom cause a headache. Only 13% of strokes are hemorrhagic, and 87% are ischemic. The distinction is important because clot-busting drugs can clear an obstruction from a cerebral artery, and may prevent brain damage if given within 3 hours of the first symptoms. So time is critical. Hospital treatment begins with a brain scan to tell whether the stroke is ischemic or hemorrhagic.

If you suspect a stroke, ask:
- When did the symptoms begin?
- Have you ever had a stroke before?
- Do you have a headache?
- Any numbness? One side or both sides?
- Any balance or vision problems?
- Any nausea or incontinence?
- Did you hit your head recently?
- Have you ever had a seizure?

To test for a stroke:
- Look for face droop on one side: Ask the patient to smile.
- Listen to the patient's speech: Is it slurred?
- Look for arm drift: Ask the patient to raise both arms; does one arm drop?
- Feel and compare the patient's grip in both hands. Is one side weaker?

Both ischemic strokes and heart attacks are caused by blockage of an artery that supplies tissues in a vital organ; so both afflictions can dramatically impair vital functions. Also, just as a heart attack may have been preceded by recurring **angina pectoris** ("pain in the chest"), an ischemic stroke may be the climax of a series of **transient ischemic attacks** (TIA), also called ministrokes. In a TIA, the symptoms subside in 24 hours or less as a clot (which may be only partially blocking the artery) is cleared away by the blood flow. But anyone who has experienced a TIA will probably have a stroke someday, without preventive treatment.

Diabetes

Since an estimated 26,000,000 diabetics live in the United States, including many whose disease has not yet been diagnosed, a diabetic emergency is one of the more likely medical problems that you may encounter on a wilderness trip. Even diabetics who can control the disease in an urban situation may run out of insulin in the wilderness, or run out of fuel because they underestimate the amount of energy they are expending. So you should know how the disease works, be able to recognize a diabetic emergency, and know what to do about it. If you are leading a wilderness trip, your medical screening of participants should include questions about diabetes, how they control it, and whether they have their insulin or other prescribed diabetic medications with them.

Metabolism and fuel delivery

The digestive system breaks down carbohydrates into a sugar (**glucose**), which is used by the body's cells for fuel. As the amount of glucose in the blood increases, it normally triggers the release of a hormone called **insulin** from the pancreas. Insulin helps transport glucose across the cell membranes and into the cells. Without insulin, glucose accumulates in the blood while the cells run on empty. Body cells (but not brain cells) have an alternative energy cycle that breaks down fatty acids, but it is much less efficient.

The pancreas also secretes **glucagon**, which raises and maintains the blood glucose level by converting stored glycogen in the liver to glucose. When the blood sugar level drops, the adrenal glands release **epinephrine**, which stops insulin secretion and increases glucose release from the liver.

If untreated, diabetes causes devastating damage all over the body, because without a dependable supply of fuel, the cells cannot do adequate maintenance and repair. Deterioration of the blood vessels increases the risk of cardiovascular disease. Deterioration of nerves can cause blindness and loss of sensation (starting in the extremities) which in turn can lead to infection of unfelt sores or wounds. So diabetics with this problem need to do frequent foot checks on hikes for blisters that could turn into open sores; and outings leaders should do this for any diabetic children. Deterioration of blood vessels in the extremities can also impede wound healing and increase the risk of infection by reducing the delivery of oxygen to the limbs (if not alleviated by hyperbaric oxygen therapy). As a result, diabetics may lose limbs to gangrene.

Types of diabetes

There are two types of diabetes. In **Type I diabetes**, the body's immune system destroys the insulin-producing cells. Many cases are associated with childhood exposure to a flu virus such as Coxsackie, which has a protein in its shell very similar to a protein on the insulin-producing cells. So antibodies produced against the virus may attack the body's own cells. Type I is called juvenile diabetes, because it usually begins early, and almost always starts in patients under 30. They tend to be thin, with weight loss and muscle wasting; and before insulin was available for medication, they did not live long. There are several types of insulin: short-acting (usually taken before meals); intermediate acting; and long acting (taken once a day). A diabetic may be taking more than one type of insulin as well as other medications.

In **Type II diabetes** (90% of all cases in the United States), the cells become **insulin-resistant**, so that it takes more and more insulin to transport glucose across cell membranes. **Hypothermia** also increases insulin resistance, with similar effects. Regular exercise, on the other hand, reduces insulin resistance. Risk factors for Type II diabetes include:

- high sugar diet;
- sedentary habits;
- obesity (increases peripheral insulin resistance);
- smoking (doubles the risk).

Type II diabetes is usually treated first with diet (especially eliminating high-sugar junk food) and exercise. Cucumbers, dill pickles, and aloe vera juice seem to be helpful in controlling blood sugar. If diet and exercise are not effective, oral medications are prescribed. If these medications are not effective, then insulin is prescribed. While Type II diabetes has traditionally been a disease of middle age or old age, it is now appearing in more and more adolescents and children, because junk food dominates their diets. The percentage of obese children in the United States has been increasing rapidly, and about 85% of Type II diabetics are obese.

Diabetic emergencies

The most common diabetic emergency is **hypoglycemia** ("too little sugar"), which means that the patient has run out of fuel. It usually comes on very suddenly. Blood sugar level is low either because it has been too long since the last meal, or because the patient took too much insulin or other diabetic medication.

Signs and symptoms usually include:
- faintness and dizziness;
- weakness;
- possible tremors.

Breathing and pulse may still be normal, or rapid. The patient may also experience:
- headache;
- double vision;
- seizures;
- apathy or irritability;
- drooling from the mouth;
- tingling or numbness in the hands and feet.

Low blood sugar triggers the release of **epinephrine**, which affects the circulatory system as well as glucose production and release, as part of the fight or flight reaction. Pulse rate may increase (tachycardia), and the skin may become pale, cool and sweaty as blood is withdrawn from the skin.

Even people who are not diabetic can suffer hypoglycemia, though it is much easier for them to restore the fuel and insulin balance. Aerobic athletes call it "hitting the wall," and can experience it either by burning all their stored (and easily metabolized) carbohydrates or by eating too much refined sugar at once and triggering an extreme insulin reaction (**rebound hypoglycemia**).

Treatment is to give a little glucose or honey and see if the patient improves. Then the patient can munch some energy food or sip a sugared drink. Diabetics may be carrying glucose self-injectors, which quickly infuse glucose directly into the thigh muscle.

Unlike other cells in the body, **brain cells** do not have an alternate fuel cycle that uses fatty acids to produce energy. They are completely dependent on a steady supply of glucose, which makes the brain extremely sensitive to hypoglycemia. When blood sugar drops too low, brain cells start to die; severe hypoglycemia is life-threatening without an immediate intake of sugar in some form.

In **hyperglycemia**, too much sugar is accumulating in the blood because there is not enough insulin to transport it into the cells, or because the cells are insulin-resistant. People who are hyperglycemic may be undiagnosed diabetics, or known diabetics who did not take their medication. Fortunately, it usually comes on slowly over a period of several hours or days. Early signs and symptoms come from the body's dumping of excess glucose in the blood through frequent urination and from lack of glucose in the cells:
- Excessive sweating (sweat may taste sweet);
- Excessive urination (physicians in earlier times diagnosed diabetes by the sweet taste of the urine);
- Excessive thirst (drinking water helps dilute the concentration of glucose in the blood);
- Weakness (from lack of glucose in the cells).

Later signs and symptoms may include:
- intense thirst and dry mouth;
- red, dry and warm skin;
- rapid deep breathing, may be rasping or sighing;
- rapid and weak pulse from dehydration;
- sunken eyes (also from dehydration);
- dim vision;
- fruity or acetone breath odor from ketones (product of less efficient fatty acid metabolism);
- confusion and disorientation;
- vomiting and abdominal pain;

Treatment is for the patient to rehydrate and take insulin, along with any other prescribed diabetic medications. If insulin is not available, you need to evacuate immediately. Meanwhile, you can reduce the level of sugar in the blood by having the patient drink as much water or unsweetened fluid as possible. However, if you are unsure whether a patient is hypo or hyperglycemic, you should always try giving sugar first. If hypoglycemia is the problem, the patient's condition should improve quickly, and you may save a life. But a little sugar will do no harm even if the patient is hyperglycemic.

Seizures

In a seizure, an uncontrolled burst of electrical activity in the brain alters consciousness and may affect muscular control. The word comes from Old French "*seisir*", which means "to take possession of," because people having seizures appeared to be possessed. Seizures range from a momentary lapse of attention or minor muscular twitches (petit mal or "little evil") to a loss of muscular control and unconsciousness.

A petit mal or **absence seizure**, which is most common in children, usually lasts just a few seconds. After a blank stare and possibly some blinking or chewing, the patient becomes alert again, and may not be aware of what happened. A **febrile seizure**, most common in children from 6 months to 6 years old, is caused by high fever, and if the seizure does not quickly subside, you need to cool the patient to prevent brain damage.

In a partial (psychomotor) seizure, which involves one cerebral hemisphere, the patient will be awake but unaware of his or her surroundings. You will see a blank stare, then random activity such as mumbling, chewing, or clumsy movement.

A generalized or grand mal ("big evil") seizure involves both cerebral hemispheres. It may start with a fall and muscular rigidity (**tonus**) that can expel air from the lungs in a loud cry; then continue with violent thrashing (**clonus**). Uncontrolled muscular contractions caused by generalized seizures are called **convulsions** (Latin *convelere*, "to pull together").

A grand mal seizure may last a minute or more. After the convulsions, the patient may lose control of bladder and bowels, may be disoriented, and may sleep for some time afterwards.

Anything that seriously disrupts brain activity can cause a seizure:
* heat stroke;
* out of control fever;
* head injury;
* not enough fuel (diabetes);
* not enough oxygen;
* hypertension;
* meningitis (several types carried by mosquitoes);
* drug or alcohol abuse;
* chronic condition (epilepsy).

Your immediate concerns in a major seizure are to:
* Protect the head and spine as the patient falls.
* Put a cushion under the head if possible.
* Protect the airway if the patient vomits – turn onto the left side and wipe away or suction vomitus.
* Clear away things that the patient could strike.
* Find out the cause, and whether you can do anything about it.

The word **epilepsy** comes from the Greek *epilepsis* "a laying hold of," because it appeared that some force or influence, presumably from the gods, had laid hold of a person having a seizure. The Romans called it *morbus sacer*, "the sacred disease." A patient with epilepsy may be carrying medication (which may not be intended for use immediately after a seizure), but is unlikely to be wearing a medic alert bracelet or necklace, because epileptics are not covered by the Americans with Disabilities Act, and could suffer discrimination with no legal recourse. Epileptics often learn to recognize the mental changes that precede a generalized seizure, and can take different forms in different people. This sense of an impending seizure is called an **aura** from the Latin word for "a breeze" (which may signal a change in weather). In Prince Myshkin, the protagonist of Dostoyevsky's novel *The Idiot*, the aura takes the form of a feeling of ecstasy and oneness with the world. An epileptic may therefore warn you of an impending seizure, and give you the chance to prepare. Dostoyevsky was an epileptic, so he was writing about seizures from his own experience.

One seizure in a known epileptic needn't end a trip, if the patient recovers well, especially if the patient is carrying medication. But a seizure with any other cause, or an unexplained seizure, usually requires rapid evacuation. A seizure that does not end (status epilepticus), or repeated seizures, will quickly become a medical emergency because the patient cannot breathe effectively when the muscles (including those that control breathing) are spasming uncontrollably.

Gastrointestinal illness

Digestion of food begins in the mouth. An enzyme in saliva begins to break down carbohydrates, and the process continues in the stomach and small intestine. Gastric juices in the stomach begin to break down proteins, but the process of digesting fats does not start until they reach the small intestine. Since the organisms that cause gastrointestinal illness (GI) generally colonize the intestine, carbohydrates will be easiest to tolerate, and fats most difficult to digest.

Dysentery (Greek "bad gut") is caused by bacteria that invade dead tissue or open sores (ulcers), usually in the large intestine. It can cause abdominal cramps and blood in the stool, though the victim may not be able to move the stool. **Diarrhea** (Greek "flowing through") is much more common and is usually caused by the body's response to toxins (Latin *toxicum* "poison") released by organisms in food or in the small intestine. The inner surface of the intestine secretes excess fluid, making the stool soft or watery. As a result, the victim becomes dehydrated, and with watery diarrhea, can soon lose enough electrolytes to cause an imbalance. If the toxin is already in the food (food poisoning), then the symptoms may begin the same day. Most organisms that colonize the intestine and produce toxins there take longer to cause symptoms.

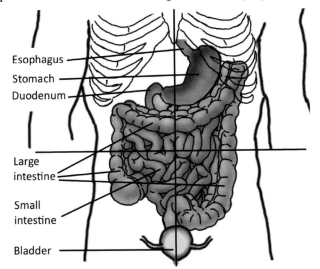

Sources of infection

Infected people and animals shed the infecting organisms in the stools, whether any symptoms are shown or not. Some organisms will remain in the stools and continue being shed long after the victim has recovered. These include Giardia and Cryptosporidium as well as some types of E. Coli. The shed organisms may then contaminate water or inadequately washed hands (fecal-oral route). In the wilderness, contaminated water is a common source of infection. Contaminated or spoiled food can also transmit infection, as well as infected people who handle food or utensils for a group. Ironically, soap on pots and dishes that have not been well rinsed can cause diarrhea. Also, about 7% of the population is sensitive enough to iodine that they may get diarrhea from using it to disinfect water.

Prevention

Water disinfection and good camp hygiene are the most important ways to prevent diarrhea in the wilderness. If you swim or bathe in contaminated water, you can accidentally swallow enough to be infected. You should also **clean your hands** thoroughly with soap and water after defecating and before handling food. If water is scarce, you can use **benzalkonium chloride** antiseptic wipes. If you carry fresh fruit and vegetables on a wilderness trip, pre-wash and dry them at home, so that you do not risk

contaminating them by washing with unsafe water. Dehydrated food is usually safe, because most bacteria that cause GI cannot grow without water.

Possible signs and symptoms

Anyone with five or more bowel movements per day, or stools that are loose or watery, has diarrhea. Other common signs and symptoms of GI are nausea, vomiting, gas, and abdominal cramps. A mild case may run its course in a day or two, but if it persists for more than two days, then the victim will probably not be able to continue the trip and should be evacuated. More serious signs and symptoms that also require evacuation are digested blood in the stools (giving it a dark, pitchy appearance), high temperature, swollen abdomen or progressive dehydration in someone who cannot replace fluid loss.

Treatment

For anyone with diarrhea, the most important treatment is fluid replacement. Water or clear fluids such as apple juice, herbal tea and clear broth (with no fat in it) are all good for mild diarrhea. For moderate or severe diarrhea, you need to replace electrolytes as well. You can use a commercial mixture (runner's drink or Oral Rehydration Salts) or make your own by adding to each liter of water:

*   1/2 teaspoon table salt (sodium chloride);
*   1/2 teaspoon baking soda;
*   1/4 teaspoon salt substitute (potassium chloride)
*   sugar or honey to taste (but not too much).

Alternate electrolyte drink with plain water. If rapid evacuation of such a patient to a hospital is not possible, you may decide to give an anti-motility agent. Check for allergies before giving any medication. Bismuth subsalicylate (Pepto-Bismol), for instance, should not be given to anyone sensitive to products that contain aspirin. Another drug, loperamide (Imodium) should not be given to children.

It is generally not safe to give anti-motility agents for diarrhea if signs and symptoms indicate a severe case, such as an oral temperature over 101° F, swollen abdomen, or blood in the stools. A patient with that serious an illness should be evacuated immediately. Antibiotics are available for many of the organisms that cause diarrhea, but the organisms need to be identified first, which requires laboratory testing.

Hydrocortisone cream (1%) can help relieve anal irritation in someone with severe diarrhea.

Recovery diet

Once the patient has started to recover, you can add simple carbohydrates in the form of crackers and toast, gelatin, and hard-boiled eggs (for easily digestible protein) to the fluid diet. When the diarrhea is nearly gone, you can add more carbohydrate foods such as boiled or baked potatoes, plain noodles, rice, bananas, and applesauce. But avoid all fatty foods and milk products as well as fruit and vegetables until the stools are normal, because they are too difficult for an impaired digestive system to digest. When the stools are normal, you can add lean meat, cooked vegetables and yogurt or cottage cheese. You should continue to avoid alcohol, spicy foods and stewed fruit for at least several days to prevent a possible relapse.

Organisms that cause intestinal disease (enteric pathogens) can be transmitted by contaminated hands, food or water. They include parasites, bacteria and viruses. Parasites may pass out of the intestine as cysts, which have tough, protective outer layers. Cysts, as well as some bacteria and viruses, can survive in water for weeks or months, even in winter. Water may also contain parasite eggs.

While the risk of infection is greatest in water that has been obviously polluted by campers, cattle or pack animals, even lakes and streams that appear pristine may be contaminated. Since the incubation period of some disease organisms may be a week or more, wilderness travelers may not always realize where they picked up an infection. However, an infection may come from contaminated food or poor group hygiene, rather than from water.

Water disinfection

Bringing water to a vigorous, roiling boil (at any altitude to which you can climb) kills all organisms that can make you sick and makes the water safe to drink. As altitude increases, the boiling temperature decreases. But as the water heats to the boiling point, it is killing microorganisms, and any temperature over 140° F. should kill them within seconds.

One device uses UV radiation to disinfect water – Hydro-Photon Steripen (www.hydrophoton.com). However, it can be used only on small quantities of water. Also, the batteries may be affected by cold weather, and any particles in the water will block some of the UV, so clarify cloudy water by straining it through a coffee filter or clean cloth.

Chemical disinfection

Chlorine and **iodine** in water may disinfect it, but several factors can interfere with the process.

- Particles in water may react with the chemicals and take them out of action; so clarify cloudy water.
- Disinfection, like any chemical reaction, depends on temperature. The colder the water, the slower the reaction. Warming water by hanging a translucent water bottle in the sun will speed the reaction.
- Giardia and Cryptosporidium cysts are most resistant to chemicals, because of their tough outer covering. But boiling easily kills them; and they are easy to filter out.

Chlorine

Halazone tablets release chlorine as they dissolve in water. But exposure to air, heat, or moisture rapidly reduces their potency, and even if they are stored in a cool, dry place, shelf life is only about six months. Moreover, chlorine is unlikely to be effective against Giardia or Cryptosporidium cysts. Many outbreaks of giardiasis have occurred in small cities with chlorinated water systems.

Iodine

Iodine also comes in tablets (Potable Aqua, Globaline, EDWGT), but these have the same problems as chlorine tablets. While sealed bottles of iodine tablets have a shelf life of four to five years, frequent opening reduces their useful life to about two weeks, so you should get a new bottle for each trip. Iodine crystals are more reliable. Adding water to the crystals makes a saturated iodine solution, which is poured into the drinking water. The **Polar Pure®** system has iodine crystals in a bottle with a thermometer on the side. Concentration of a saturated iodine solution depends on its temperature.

Recommended doses of iodine are calculated for a temperature of 68° to 77° F. In a transparent bottle, you can tell how saturated the solution is by its color. Pale yellow is weak and dark orange is strong. If the solution is weak, you can warm it up next to your body. Let it equilibrate for 30 to 60 minutes before using, or increase the dose by 30%.

Doses from a 2 oz. bottle are usually given in bottle caps. One capful holds 2.5 cc. For clear water, use five caps of the solution. Be careful not to let any crystals into the water bottle. Shake the bottle well. You should allow at least 15 minutes contact time if water is warm or 60 minutes if it is cold. For cloudy water, use ten caps of solution. Allow 30 minutes if the water is warm or 60 minutes if it is cold.

Alcohol solutions of iodine also work. For 2% tincture of iodine, just substitute one drop for each capful of the water solution and allow the same contact times. For 10% Povidone/iodine solution (Betadyne), use eight drops instead of five capfuls, sixteen drops instead of ten capfuls. You can also add 100 cc of 95% ethanol to 8 grams of iodine crystals. Just 1 cc of the ethanol solution equals five capfuls of the water solution. CAUTION: use only U.S.D.A. food-grade resublimated iodine crystals. Other iodine crystals for industrial use contain impurities that may be toxic.

About 7% of the population may have a reaction to iodine, usually diarrhea. Iodine is not recommended for pregnant women or people with thyroid problems. Also, the longer you use it the more likely you are to have problems. So on a long trip, iodine is probably best reserved as a backup to other disinfection techniques, such as boiling or filtering.

Making the water palatable

You can remove the taste of iodine by sprinkling vitamin C crystals in the water or using a powdered drink flavoring that includes vitamin C (ascorbic acid). Be careful not to do this until disinfection is complete because it will inactivate the iodine. It will not, however, remove iodine. To do that, you would need to run the water through a block of granular activated carbon, available as an attachment on some filters.

Water filters

Intake hoses attached to water filters usually have screens to keep out large particles, and there may be one or more pre-filters. But the **absolute size** of the pores in the final filter tells you what size organisms the filter can remove. "Absolute" means that all pores are that size or smaller. micron) pore size may be 0.4μ

absolute pore size. So be sure that the specifications refer to absolute (not **nominal**) pore size.

A filter must have an absolute pore size of 0.2μ to remove bacteria as well as larger organisms. Viruses are about 0.01μ, much too small for filtration in the field. While many of them will be removed because they tend to clump or attach to larger particles, some will get through. Some filters use an iodine resin matrix to kill any organisms that pass through the filter. This element may be built into the filter or sold as an optional attachment. Filters with an iodine matrix remove viruses almost completely, though in some tests they do not quite meet the Environmental Protection Agency standard of removing 99.99%.

Some filters include a block of granular activated carbon, which may remove chemicals, such as pesticide from agricultural runoff, or the residue from chemical disinfection.

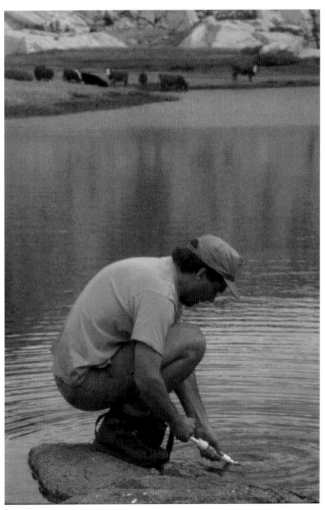

Hiker using a filter on suspect water. Note the cows across the lake. *Photos courtesy of Ben Schifrin, MD*

Filter types

Filters are of two types: **membrane** and **labyrinth**. Membrane filters are thin and delicate and cannot be cleaned, so you need to carry replacements, especially on a long trip. Labyrinth filters are solid structures that can be cleaned. The pores are twisting paths through the thickness of the filter, so the filter element would have to be seriously damaged to fail. It is also harder for organisms to get through than a thin membrane with the same pore size.

Ceramic filter elements (used in some Katadyn and MSR filters) last at least ten times as long as the others and can be brushed off when they get clogged, so they have an advantage on long trips. But how resistant are they to damage? They are also brittle, so they could be cracked if dropped or if frozen with water inside. The **borosilicate labyrinth filter** used in the Sweetwater Guardian, and the **pleated glass fiber** used in PUR and other filters are rugged, and also cleanable, though they will not last as long as ceramic filters. Several manufacturers also make **gravity filters**, which can be useful in a base camp where you have time to let the water slowly seep through.

Convenience

How easy and convenient are the filters to use? The Katadyn Pocket filter is the hardest and most awkward to pump, because you have to brace it against something solid when you depress the piston. The SweetWater and the MSR filters, with lever handles, are the easiest to pump. Some filters have adapters on the outlet hose that fit standard water bottles.

How easy are the filters to maintain? The MSR filters are very well designed. The Waterworks II has four filter elements of decreasing size, which greatly reduces clogging. But it must be taken apart regularly to clean and dry out, and includes a number of small parts that can be misplaced. So it tends to be popular with people who are mechanically adept and don't mind doing regular maintenance. Most other filters seem to require little maintenance.

Poisoning

If food is contaminated with an organism that has already produced toxins, they will not be inactivated by cooking. They can make you sick in less than seven hours. Some examples of bacteria whose toxins can cause food poisoning are Staphylococcus aureus, Salmonella, Shigella, and Clostridium botulinum. **Staphylococcus** can grow even in food cured with salt, such as ham that has not been kept refrigerated. **Salmonella** is common in poultry and sometimes in eggs, because most poultry feed is augmented with protein from slaughterhouse products. It can also be found in meat and unpasteurized dairy products. The bacteria in poultry intestines contaminate the carcasses and the outside of the eggs. Most adults in the United States probably have some degree of immunity from Salmonella, because the incidence in humans drops very steeply from the age of one to the age of nine. **Shigella** is often transmitted by flies as well as infected food handlers. **Clostridium botulinum** can be found in canned as well as raw food, especially fish. Since it is anaerobic, it does not need oxygen, so it can grow and produce toxin inside a can with contaminated food.

Signs and symptoms

All food poisoning upsets the digestive process and can cause nausea and vomiting as well as diarrhea and sometimes abdominal cramps. With Salmonella toxin, the diarrhea is often foul and watery, and the victim may also get a headache. **Botulism** is especially dangerous, because after several days of gastro-intestinal upset, it can attack the nervous system. The victim may experience dry mouth and hoarseness, difficulty swallowing, facial weakness, sluggish pupils, blurred or double vision, and muscular weakness that can progress into paralysis. If untreated, it is often fatal, but there is an antitoxin for it. So if you suspect botulism, it is important to get the victim to a hospital where it can be diagnosed and treated before it attacks the nervous system.

Other poisoning routes

Most poisons are ingested; but they can also be inhaled, absorbed through skin or mucus membranes, or injected (see chapters 25 and 26 on venomous bites and stings). The word poison comes from the Latin *potio* "potion" by way of the early French *puison*. To the Romans, *potio* also meant a magical drink. In English, a poison is any substance that causes harm when it gets inside the body, by either destroying cells or disrupting their functions.

Poisoning information and treatment

Any business that uses potentially toxic chemicals should have **Material Safety Data Sheets** (MSDS) that describe the hazards, how to protect yourself, and what to do if you are exposed. But if you have phone reception, you can call the **American Association of Poison Control Centers** (www.aapcc.org) at their 24-hour hotline: 1-800-222-1222. Their staff gives expert advice on what to do after exposure to any poison.

Inducing vomiting is no longer recommended for ingested poisons, because the vomitus can be aspirated into the lungs (especially if the patient is less than fully alert) and corrosive poisons that caused direct damage going down would do even more damage coming up. But **activated charcoal** is recommended for some poisons if the patient is alert enough to swallow safely. It is a fine black powder that adsorbs (binds to) poisons in the stomach and intestines, so that they pass through the digestive system instead of being absorbed into the blood. But it does not work on corrosive poisons (such as drain cleaner) or alcohol.

Ingested and absorbed poisons

Overdosing on drugs, which can be over the counter, prescription, or recreational is a common cause of poisoning. Symptoms (which may be delayed as the drug moves through the digestive system and into the blood) may include abdominal pain, nausea, vomiting, or diarrhea. Overdoses of drugs designed to bring vital functions into the normal range can be especially dangerous. For example, too much of an anti-clotting drug can cause internal bleeding. Overdoses of many medications can affect the heart rate, blood pressure, or breathing as well as the level of responsiveness. Overdoses of depressants (including alcohol, barbiturates and narcotics) can cause respiratory arrest.

Many plants are poisonous, including ornamental plants in gardens and houses as well as those found in the wilderness. Many household products are very poisonous if swallowed. For example, pesticides are designed to kill plants or vermin, so they are very toxic to humans; and cleaning products usually have corrosive ingredients. The oil in poison oak, ivy, and sumac can be absorbed through the skin, and so can any poisons (such as pesticides) that are mixed in liquid solvents.

Inhaled poisons

Volatile chemicals (Latin *volatilis* "flying") have a very low boiling point, so even at room temperature some of the liquid evaporates into fumes. A reaction from mixing chemicals can also produce fumes. For example, mixing ammonia and bleach produces chlorine gas. Some other household products that produce toxic fumes are oven, toilet bowl and drain cleaners; oil-based paint; paint thinner; and bug foggers or sprays. Combustion (burning), a chemical reaction that releases heat, can also release toxic gases as well as particles that cause inhalation injury.

Probably the most common and insidious inhaled poison is carbon monoxide, which is odorless. **Carbon monoxide** is produced by incomplete combustion of any material containing carbon, and is found in the smoke from house and forest fires as well as fumes from cooking with petroleum-based or natural gas fuel. So it is a hazard of cooking in tents and snow caves (see chapter 7). Carbon monoxide is also a component of automobile exhaust and a potential hazard in buildings using natural gas for heating, which should have carbon monoxide detectors with alarms. Carbon monoxide binds to hemoglobin much more strongly than oxygen, so it reduces the oxygen carrying capacity of the blood. **Hydrogen cyanide** is also odorless. It is produced from burning fabrics, paper, plastics and other synthetics that are common in modern buildings. Hydrogen cyanide prevents cells from using oxygen.

Symptoms of hypoxia from carbon monoxide poisoning vary and are similar to symptoms of many other conditions: headache, nausea, tachycardia (Greek *tachys* "swift" + *kardia* "heart"), possible seizure, and unconsciousness. Symptoms of hydrogen cyanide poisoning in low doses may include headache, vertigo, drowsiness, tachycardia, and tachypnea ("swift breathing").

Victims of moderate or high doses may experience tremors, cardiac arrhythmia (irregular heartbeat), convulsions, stupor and paralysis, as well as respiratory depression. Immediate treatment for both carbon monoxide and hydrogen cyanide exposure is **oxygen administration.**

Pregnancy and Wilderness Activity

Pregnant women breathe and circulate blood for two. If they are in good aerobic condition, they will be able to meet these demands more easily. During labor and delivery, when the mother's own demand for blood and oxygen increases, aerobic fitness provides an extra safety margin, which helps keep the baby well oxygenated.

Muscle tone is also important during pregnancy. Pregnant women carry considerable extra weight, whose distribution puts stress on back, abdominal, and leg muscles. Strong and well-exercised muscles make it easier to adapt to this stress. Mothers with good muscle tone are also likely to find labor easier, especially the second stage and the afterbirth, when they use their abdominal muscles to push. Pregnant women who have been sedentary, however, should begin exercise like walking gradually and not try to reach a high level of aerobic fitness during pregnancy. Maintaining a level of fitness to which your body is accustomed is much easier than getting in condition; and the developing fetus places an aerobic demand on the mother's heart and lungs even at rest.

Pregnant women need to guard against two hazards which can bring on pre-term labor: dehydration, and urinary tract infection. Pre-term labor in the first four months of pregnancy usually results in a miscarriage (spontaneous abortion).

Vital signs in pregnancy

Plasma volume (the liquid part of the blood) increases by up to 40% which increases blood volume; and the number of red blood cells also increases if the mother's diet includes adequate iron, which increases oxygen carrying capacity. Stroke volume (the amount of blood pushed out of the ventricles with each contraction) increases and the heart beats more rapidly to move more blood through the system each minute. A resting pulse rate of 70 before pregnancy may increase to 100 by the third trimester, and be as high as 120 when the woman goes into labor. Blood pressure, however, should not be increased by pregnancy, and may become somewhat lower by the third trimester

A rise of 30 mm Hg or more in her systolic blood pressure, or 15 mm Hg or more in her diastolic blood pressure, may be a sign of **preeclampsia**, a potentially life-threatening condition that can begin after the twentieth week. In preeclampsia, blood flow to the kidneys is disrupted, causing water and salt retention, so another sign of preeclampsia is **edema**. Symptoms may include headache, blurred vision, and abdominal pain. Diabetes and pre-existing hypertension seem to be risk factors.

Pregnant women breathe more deeply even at rest, to satisfy the additional oxygen demands of the fetus. Tidal volume (the amount of air moved in and out of the lungs with each breath) increases up to 40% by the third trimester. But the respiratory rate usually does not increase, and an abnormal rate of breathing is cause for concern. Also, if breathing is depressed, it is important to give oxygen promptly because more than one life may be at stake.

Activity and hydration

It is easy to become dehydrated during wilderness activity. Pregnant women must be especially careful to drink enough, because dehydration can cause pre-term labor. During pregnancy, they should drink at least two liters of water per day, plus enough to replace what they lose by excess sweating. Severe dehydration decreases blood volume, and blood pressure increases to compensate. They must also be careful to take in electrolytes when they are drinking water. Electrolyte imbalance can cause fluid shift out of blood vessels, which will also decrease blood volume.

Infection

Both **urinary tract infection** (UTI) and vaginal infection can cause pre-term labor. **Vaginal infection** may cause itching, which a pregnant woman should report promptly to her obstetrician or midwife. It can be caused by sexually transmitted organisms (e.g., gonorrhea) or by an imbalance in organisms normally present. For **urinary tract infection**, see chapter 28 (Medical emergencies in the wilderness).Pregnant women should have a UTI treated immediately, and if they have a history of UTIs, carry their prescription medication for UTI with them on wilderness trips.

Chapter 9. Wilderness first aid kits

Many people who do wilderness activities give little thought to first aid kits, until they learn – the hard way – that they are not prepared to deal with wilderness accidents. Emergency care training should give you some skill at improvising. But without the proper equipment, you will be handicapped at best, and at worst, you'll find yourself unable to treat injuries effectively or prevent complications.

For practical purposes, injuries are of three types: those that will kill the victim unless something is done immediately; those that cause serious damage and that may kill or disable the victim in time; and minor injuries, which would normally cause only temporary discomfort. In the wilderness, however, even minor injuries like foot blisters can be disabling. And keep in mind that infections are much more of a hazard when you are far from help, since they have more time to develop and become dangerous.

Wounds, dressings and bandages

Anything that stops breathing or circulation will kill within minutes at normal body temperature. In these situations, a first aid kit may not be of much help. To control serious arterial bleeding, which can also kill within a few minutes, you need a bulky dressing and something to hold it in place.

For most bleeding wounds, 4" x 4" sterile gauze pads work well. For severe bleeding, surgical dressings (trauma pads) are very absorbent, with a non-stick layer to cover the wound.

Triangular (cravat) bandages are very versatile. They can apply strong pressure on a bleeding wound, as well as holding a dressing in place; and if direct pressure does not work, they can be used as tourniquets. Triangular bandages can be bought, or made, by cutting a piece of fabric (perhaps an old bed sheet) at least 40" square, on the diagonal. This will give you two triangular bandages. Hem the cut edges and you have two deluxe triangular bandages.

Rolls of stretchy gauze are good for general wrapping – the 4" width seems to be most useful, and 2" rolls are good for finger bandages. You should also have two rolls of tape: a narrow (1/2" - 3/4") roll of porous athletic tape, which can hold dressings in place without cutting off air flow; and a 2" roll of duct tape.

A good selection of band aids will cover most small wounds. For wounds in which bleeding is not a problem, non-stick pads on the dressings are best.

Butterfly closures are often used even by doctors to close gaping cuts, as an alternative to the traumatic technique of suturing. These sterile adhesive strips with narrow bridges in the center hold wounds shut without pressing on them. Superglue has long been used by trainers to close cuts on boxers, and there are formulations made for wound closure.

Disinfecting and cleaning agents

Antiseptics like povidone-iodine and benzalkonium chloride are sold in foil packets as well as bottles. Use the liquid form, which will spread through the wound area, not the ointment. A container of honey, however, would be a better addition to your first aid kit.

Irrigating a wound effectively requires a forceful jet of water (7-8 psi) to flush out debris. A wound irrigation syringe with a blunt needle will do the job best. A plastic squeeze bottle with a screw-on cap and a very narrow nozzle will also produce a forceful stream. Squeezing a ziplock bag with a pinhole in a bottom corner will produce about 2 psi of pressure.

Use biodegradable liquid soap to wash your hands before treating a wound. In the absence of water, benzalkonium chloride antiseptic pads can do a reasonable job of cleaning your hands as well as the skin around a wound – but remember to wipe away from the wound!

Gloves help to protect you and your patient from sharing infections. Synthetic gloves, such as nitrile, avoid the danger of latex allergy in you or your patient.

Fractures and splints

Splints can be improvised from poles, ice axes, the staves of internal-frame backpacks, rolled-up foam pads – anything that will support and immobilize the fractured limb. Splinting is easier, however, with a splint designed for the job.

- SAM splints (www.sammedical.com) designed by an orthopedist, are thin strips of flexible aluminum (4.25" by 36") with foam on both sides. It weighs 4 oz. and rolls or folds up compactly.
- You can make a wire splint by cutting a 6" piece off a 30" roll of hardware cloth (1/4" wire mesh, available at a hardware store). Trim the projecting wires from the cut edges and cover them with duct tape. This kind of splint functions like a SAM, but needs padding.

To hold splints in place, you can use cravat, gauze roller, or elastic bandages. You can also secure them with duct tape, though that would make it difficult to adjust the tension when the fractured limb swells. For an arm fracture, a triangular bandage will make a sling, though you can improvise with the bottom of the patient's shirt or jacket – fold it up to cradle the arm and safety pin it together. Even without a splint, this will help stabilize a fractured arm.

In freezing weather, the hand or foot of a fractured limb is very vulnerable to frostbite. Damage to blood vessels by the broken bone ends, constriction by splint fasteners, and the victim's inability to move the splinted limb all tend to interfere with circulation. In this case, one or two hand warmers, well wrapped and secured, may be the only way to keep the extremity from freezing. Cheap, disposable warmers weigh less than 3 ounces and give up to 20 hours of heat.

Medications

You can avoid most discomforts that might tempt you to use medications in the back country by taking care of yourself: putting enough water and fuel into your system; disinfecting drinking water; acclimatizing and dressing properly. Used with caution, however, medications can prevent a trip from becoming an ordeal, and free you from distracting discomfort.

Aspirin and ibuprofen are anti-inflammatory as well as analgesic (pain-killing). These medications may be needed for burns and wear-and-tear injuries, which involve swelling or inflammation, especially in heavily used joints like the knees. Enteric-coated aspirin are more durable, and less likely to cause stomach irritation. Tylenol (acetaminophen with codeine) is a stronger medication for relieving moderate pain. Codeine is an oral narcotic for relieving severe pain.

Antihistamines or decongestants may help if narrowing or clogging of the air passages makes breathing and sleeping difficult. Epinephrine, in an inhaler or epipen, might save the life of a victim with a severe allergic reaction to insect venom or other foreign protein by opening constricted breathing passages.

Gastrointestinal miseries, though usually preventable, are debilitating and common. A laxative can relieve constipation. An oral rehydration mix with electrolytes can keep the victim hydrated while the disease runs its course.

For infections on a long trip, an oral antibiotic may be a lifesaver. For altitude illness, acetazolamide or dexamethasone may help. Hydrocortisone cream relieves itching, and oil of cloves can ease toothache. For a long trip, a dental first aid kit is a good idea. Anti-fungal powder or ointment will help to control athlete's foot and other fungal infections.

Prescription medications (Rx) must be obtained from a physician, for one's personal use. For a long trip, the leader can give participants a list of types of medications to get from their own physicians, e.g., oral antibiotics, to avoid the medical risk of giving people drugs to which they may be allergic, and the legal risk of practicing medicine without a license.

Pills have expiration dates on them because it is required by law. If the exact dose is critical, as with a prescription medication for a chronic illness, then these expiration dates are important. Other pills, however, can generally be used until they crumble, although they may lose some of their potency with time.

Tools

For a pocket kit, you can make do with the tiny scissors on your Swiss Army knife. A larger kit, however, should include a set of universal shears (also called paramedic or EMT shears), available from medical supply stores and some hardware suppliers. They are offset, self-sharpening bandage scissors made of stainless steel, with plastic-covered grips large enough for your whole hand. The tip of the bottom blade is blunted to slide harmlessly on skin.

If you do need to take apart clothing, it will be easier to stitch it together again if you open the seams with a seam-ripper (which you can find with other sewing supplies) rather than shredding the fabric.

Safety pins can hold the clothing together until it is repaired. Diaper pins are the strongest safety pins.

Sterilized in a flame, a needle from your sewing kit can be used to remove splinters, but Uncle Bill's Sliver Grippers are designed for the job. Short and broad, they are easy to manipulate and come to a sharp point, so that you can grip and pull out even tiny hairs of metal or fiberglass. They can also be used to remove ticks that are attached to the skin. Tick Spoon and Tick Pliers are more specialized tools that can be used to grip a tick and pull it out.

Needle nose vise grips can be used to remove large cactus spines, as well as for equipment repair. To remove tiny, hair-like spines and nettles from the skin, spread rubber cement over them, let it set, and peel it off. If you lack rubber cement, you can use duct tape.

Snakebite kits seldom help, and can cause serious damage if they require people to make incisions. Plastic suction pumps, such as Sawyer's Extractor, do not require incisions, but there is no published evidence that they actually extract venom.

A CPR mask will protect against infection when doing mouth-to-mouth respiration. For a small first aid kit, a disposable mask is the most compact. It will fit in a shirt pocket or on a key chain.

Containers

You will need a container for your kit. Before selecting it, ask what it needs to do. Must it be rigid to resist crushing, or would a flexible container be easier to pack? Must it be completely waterproof? Must it float (e.g., for rafting or boating)? A small, personal kit can go in a transparent plastic envelope with a zipper or a small freezette container secured with a nylon strap.

Another option is a nylon zipper bag with compartments, preferably the kind that folds out when opened so that all your equipment is easily accessible. For a large expedition, a military surplus ammunition box (available in three sizes) makes an almost indestructible container. Any large kit should be organized into smaller modules in labeled containers, so you can select the modules needed for a trip, and quickly find things in an emergency.

Small ziplock bags can organize and protect dressings, bandages, and other small items. Small transparent plastic screw-top containers organize pills. For liquids, such as disinfecting solution, buy plastic squeeze bottles with squirt caps (1 or 2 oz. size for small kits). Wrap the threads of the bottles with PTFE thread seal tape (available in plumbing supply sections of hardware stores) before screwing on the caps, so that they will not leak.

Survival

Equipment for personal survival may also help your patient survive. If you have to bivouac or do a long evacuation, protection against the elements may be more important than emergency care. For survival, you may need spare clothing, shelter-building supplies, fire-starters, and spare sunglasses. To find your way out or attract help, you may need a compass, watch, maps, signal mirror, whistle, and coins for a phone. A GPS can pinpoint your location, but you always need backup navigation tools in case the GPS fails, or your lines of sight to the satellites are blocked by the terrain. To transport a patient, you may need materials for building a litter or sled.

Putting it all together

A good pharmacy will have many of the supplies you need. Backpacking stores often stock wilderness-oriented items. For some items, you may have to go to a medical supply store or online catalog. Putting your own kit together (rather than buying a prepackaged kit) helps ensure that it will contain what you need. Having adequate first aid equipment and training will help you to handle emergencies quickly and efficiently so that you can then turn your attention to surviving (and even enjoying) the rest of the trip.

List of supplies

Some of the items in this list may be kept in your repair kit or elsewhere. What you pack and how much depends on trip length, activity, terrain, and number of people. If you repackage medications, copy both the expiration date and dosage information onto the new label and cover it with transparent tape for protection. Note, however, that pills can generally be used until they disintegrate, unless the exact dosage is critical. Bold face items in the list are the most versatile and essential.

Tools
Swiss Army knife or multi- tool – *Cutting, equipment repair*
EMT shears: *Cutting bandages, clothing, etc.*
Seam ripper: *Opening clothing to expose injuries*
Uncle Bill's Sliver Grippers: *Removing slivers and wound debris, can also be used to remove ticks*
Tick Spoon or Tick Pliers: *Removing ticks*
Needle nose vise grips: *Equipment repair, gripping needles*
Safety pins: *Fastening bandages, closing ripped seams*
Sewing kit with button and carpet thread: *Repair of clothing, sleeping bags, tents, packs, etc.*
Small flashlight: *Checking light response in patient's pupils, doing assessment in the dark*
Small magnifier: *Removing slivers or ticks*
Pencil or pen
Notepad
Hand/body warmers
CPR mask (small disposable one)
Cotton-tipped applicators
Mini marshmallows: *Removing contact lenses,*
Rubber cement: *Removing cactus needles and nettles*

Containers
Vinyl zipper envelope or small freezette container: *Personal kit*
Nylon zipper bags with compartments: *Group kit*
Ammo boxes: *Expedition kit*
Ziplock bags: *Organize items*
Small plastic bottles: *Organize pills*
Squeeze bottles: *Liquids, e.g. disinfectant*

Cleaning and disinfecting
Nitrile gloves (non-allergenic))
Liquid soap
Honey: *Disinfecting*
Povidone iodine (liquid): *Disinfecting*
Benzalkonium chloride prep pads: *Cleaning and disinfecting hands, skin around wound*
Syringe with blunt needle or equivalent: *Wound irrigation cleansing*

Dressings and bandages
Sterile gauze pads: *Wound dressings*
Trauma pads/battle dressings: *Bleeding control*
Band Aids (non-stick): *Wound protection*
Adhesive pads (non-stick): *Wound protection*
Triangular bandages: *Securing dressings and splints*

Gauze rollers (4"): *Securing dressings or splints*
Gauze rollers (2"): *Finger bandages*
Bias cut stockinette: *Securing dressings*
Butterfly bandages: *Wound closure*
Knuckle bandages
Fingertip bandages
Eye patch
Moleskin: *Blister prevention and treatment*
Mole foam: *Blister prevention and treatment*
2nd Skin: *Blister and burn treatment*
Athletic tape (3/4")
Duct tape: *Quick securing of splints, equipment repair*

Splints
Wire splints
SAM splints
Air splints
Traction splint: *For fractured femur*

Medications
Aspirin: *Mild pain & inflammation*
Ibuprofen: *Mild pain*
Rx Tylenol: *Moderate pain*
Rx Codeine: *Severe pain*
Antihistamine: *Allergy/asthma*
Rx Epinephrine inhaler: *Severe asthma or anaphylactic reaction*
Rx pseudoephedrine: *Decongestant*
Laxative: *For constipation*
Rx Lomotil: *For diarrhea*
Electrolyte mix: *Rehydration*
Rx erythromycin: *Moderate infection*
Rx ampicillin or cephalexin: *Severe infection*
Hydrocortisone cream (1%): Relieve itching
Oil of cloves: *Ease toothache*
Cavit dental filling paste: *Temporary filling*
Antifungal powder/ointment
Lip balm

Survival
Steel mirror and whistle: *Signaling*
Shelter or materials to make it
Extra clothing
Fire starters
Emergency food and water disinfecting system
Sun, insect protection

Recommended reading

Wilderness Emergency Care, Revised Edition. Steve Donelan. National association for Search and Rescue, 2018. This is my comprehensive guide to preventing, and coping with wilderness emergencies, on which the much shorter *Wilderness First Aid* book is based.

Wilderness Medicine, 7th Ed. Elsevier, Inc. 2017 (www.elsivierhealth.com). Ed. P.S. Auerbach. Now in two volumes, this is the only comprehensive book on the subject, with over 5,000 large, double-column pages, lavishly illustrated. Its 126 chapters (some of them as long as small books) discuss hazards, injuries, and medical problems in all outdoor environments, from the mountains to the ocean, and from the arctic to the jungle. There are also chapters on survival in and rescue from different environments; children, women, and elders in the wilderness; improvisation; the changing environment; helpful and harmful plants; and ethics of wilderness medicine. Discussion of field medical treatment is thorough. This is a one-volume library for wilderness responders and instructors, written by experts, with all the details that other books omit; and it now comes with access to a dedicated web site for references and other resources. I have used all six previous editions of this book extensively in my teaching and writing for many years.

Wilderness Medical Society: Practice Guidelines for Wilderness Emergency Care, 5th Ed., ed. William W. Forgey. Falcon Guides, 2006. This concise book is a consensus of wilderness medicine experts on how to assess and treat injuries and medical problems in the wilderness. Most instructors of wilderness emergency care courses use it for reference. I am a contributor and peer reviewer. Updated guidelines are available online at www.wms.org.

Medicine for Mountaineering and Other Wilderness Activities, 6th Ed, ed. James A. Wilkerson. The Mountaineers, 2010. Since 1935, mountaineering physicians have been teaching backcountry first aid and medicine to other mountaineers in Washington. They explain topics rather than just dispensing information, and the style is consistently clear and readable. As the title suggests, the book is mostly for mountaineers, though this edition adds more on other environments.

Medicine for the Outdoors: The Essential Guide to First Aid and Medical Emergencies, 5th Ed. Paul S. Auerbach, M.D. Mosby, 2009. Dr. Auerbach's book includes detailed information about tropical, desert, and underwater environments – he is an enthusiastic scuba diver. It has long sections on wild plant poisoning, marine hazards, and diseases in the backcountry. Dense with information and advice, it is designed more for reference than for continuous reading.

Going Higher: Oxygen, Man, and Mountains, 4th ed. Charles S. Houston, M.D. Little, Brown & Co., 1999. Dr. Houston studied the effects of altitude for over 60 years. *Going High* (1981) distilled a lifetime of research, experience, and enthusiasm into a lively and well-illustrated book, which the author revised and expanded for the third time in 1999. He also tells the fascinating story of human experience with altitude and the attempts to explain its effects.

Wilderness & Environmental Medicine, the quarterly journal of the Wilderness Medical Society features technical articles based on original research, review articles, book reviews, and abstracts of relevant articles from other journals. I edit a regular column for it called The Wilderness Instructor. All issues except the current one are freely accessible online at the Society's web site: www.wms.org.

Wilderness Search and Rescue, Tim J. Setnicka. Appalachian Mountain Club, 1981. More than 600 pages long, this book gives clear and practical instructions for performing rescues in all types of wilderness situations. The author is a park ranger who started his Search and Rescue career doing big wall rescues in Yosemite. His book is also available as a Kindle edition.

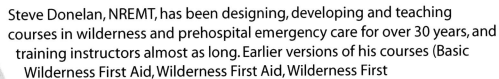

Steve Donelan, NREMT, has been designing, developing and teaching courses in wilderness and prehospital emergency care for over 30 years, and training instructors almost as long. Earlier versions of his courses (Basic Wilderness First Aid, Wilderness First Aid, Wilderness First Responder, and Wilderness EMT Upgrade) have been available through other organizations, but they are now supported by the National Association for Search and Rescue. Steve has a BA in Philosophy and Greek from the University of California, Berkeley, and did years of graduate studies in the history of science. He has published over 60 articles on emergency care and how to teach it, as well as several textbooks. He has been an instructor of the National Ski Patrol's Outdoor Emergency Care course since the beginning of the program, and is a peer reviewer of the OEC textbook. He is also the section editor and columnist on education for *Wilderness and Environmental Medicine* (journal of the Wilderness Medical Society), a peer reviewer of their *Practice Guidelines for Wilderness Emergency Care*, and a recipient of their Education Award.

Steve can be contacted about teaching and instructor training through his web site:

www.wildernessemergencycare.com.

Made in the USA
Las Vegas, NV
05 February 2024

85340474R00069